RAYNAUD'S
A guide for health professionals

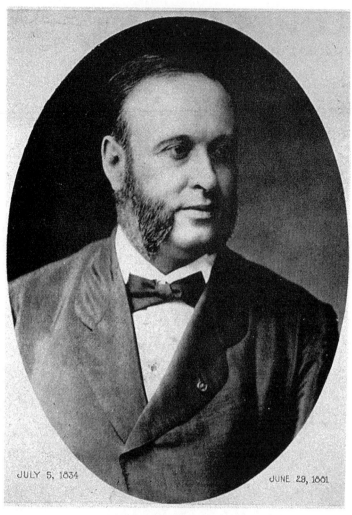

JULY 5, 1834   JUNE 29, 1881

Maurice Raynaud

RAYNAUD'S
A guide for health professionals

Edited by

STUART ROATH

Haematology
University of Southampton Medical School
For and on behalf of The Raynaud's Association

London   New York
CHAPMAN AND HALL

First published in 1989 by
Chapman and Hall Ltd
11 New Fetter Lane, London EC4P 4EE

Typeset in 10/12 Palatino
by Acorn Bookwork, Salisbury, Wiltshire
Printed in Great Britain by
St. Edmundsbury Press Ltd
Bury St. Edmunds, Suffolk

ISBN 0 412 33680 4

British Library Cataloguing in Publication Data

Raynaud's: a guide for health
   professionals.
   1. Raynaud's phenomenon
   I. Roath, S. (Stuart)
   616.1

   ISBN 0–412–33680–4

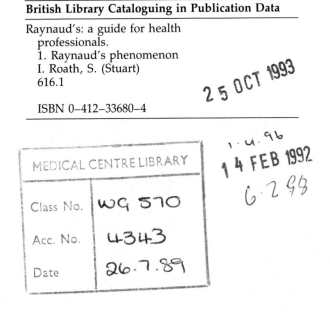

Contents

Contributors

Anne Mawdsley

Director,
The Raynaud's Association
112 Crewe Road, Alsager,
Cheshire ST7 2JA

Stuart Roath MD FRC Path FI Biol

University Haematology
Southampton General Hospital
Southampton SO9 4XY
UK

John Francis PhD
and
Deborah Francis FMILT

University Haematology
Southampton General Hospital
Southampton SO9 4XY
UK

Derek Waller DM

Clinical Pharmacology Group,
Southampton General Hospital
Southampton SO9 4XY
UK

Vivian Challenor MRCP

Clinical Pharmacology Group
Southampton General Hospital
Southampton SO9 4XY
UK

Raj Mani PhD

Medical Physics
Southampton General Hospital
Southampton SO9 4XY
UK

Robert Hayward BSc
and
Michael Griffin PhD

Human Factor Unit
Institute of Sound and Vibration
Research
University of Southampton
Southampton SO2 1TL

Ray Clark MD

Thermographics Unit
Clinical Research Centre
Watford Road
Harrow HA1 3UJ
UK

Robert Freedman PhD
Behavioral Medicine Laboratory
Wayne State University
Detroit
USA M1 48207

Foreword

This book has been published in association with The Raynaud's Association in order to give a better understanding of the condition and information regarding research and current treatments available. It has been written by doctors and research workers who are experts in this field. It is intended as a guide for members of the medical profession and workers in different branches of health care as well as social workers who may come into contact with Raynaud's sufferers.

The Raynaud's Association was formed in 1982. It was felt that there was a lack of communication between patients, most of whom felt isolated, having not met others with similar problems and many were feeling depressed. Throughout the country there appeared to be very little coordination between consultants, researchers and general practitioners, who may see only a few, if any, severe cases in their practices. Raynaud's patients were frequently being told they would have to learn to live with their condition as nothing could be done. Help and advice were seldom offered and it was difficult to find suitable information or reading material on the subject.

The aims of the Association are to promote a greater understanding and awareness of the condition, to help people to help themselves by exchanging ideas found to be useful and to raise money for research. As with all self-help groups, members usually find it is a great comfort to contact others who understand their problems. Quarterly newsletters are issued giving news of research, treatments available, advice on aids which help daily living, fund-raising ideas and achievements – as well as supplying other relevant material.

The Association has also published a book entitled *Raynaud's – A Better Understanding* by Mr K. Lafferty, MS, FRCS which has been written for patients as well as others interested in the care and welfare of sufferers of this painful and often misunderstood condition. In addition there are two patient handbooks on Raynaud's and Scleroderma which give advice to patients on how to help themselves and a booklet containing over 100 questions and answers on Raynaud's and associated conditions. The Association produce leaflets on Raynaud's, systemic sclerosis, erythromelalgia, vibration white finger and keeping warm. A patient video has been made by the Association, details of which can be sent on request.

We are most fortunate in the support we receive from doctors who are prepared to act as medical and scientific advisors. Through this close contact with the medical profession, the Association is able to advise members and their doctors on the many problems which arise. During the past few years the Association has been able to finance a substantial amount of research and is continuing to do so.

As yet it is not known how widespread the problem is but it is believed to affect one-fifth of the population, women being affected nine times more than men. There is no known cure for this condition and treatment remains the most challenging problem.

Doctors and scientists throughout the world are now taking a great deal of interest in Raynaud's and real advances have been made over the past few years.

Investigation of all diseases and conditions which are known to be associated with Raynaud's phenomenon is essential if we are to determine the common underlying pathophysiological nature of this problem, which so often results in permanent disability and loss of fingers and toes in otherwise fit adults.

The chances of finding cures are directly proportional to the amount of research we can support. The Raynaud's Association is working hard to maintain the projects which are currently underway, and even more funds are needed if this vital research programme is to be expanded.

We are indebted to Dr Stuart Roath and the contributors of this book for providing an indepth understanding of the condition.

Anne H. Mawdsley
Director
The Raynaud's Association

Preface

Raynaud's – the disease, the phenomenon, the syndrome – gives rise to considerable discomfort or even incapacity in a number of adolescents and adults in any part of the world where cold winters are the norm. Most of those affected are women and because the primary form of Raynaud's is not as spectacular as many other disorders, nor does it end fatally, the definition and investigation of this problem has been somewhat under-pursued until recently. The emergence of a national association for the disorder in the United Kingdom and many smaller associations in other parts of the world has changed this and considerable efforts are being made to define as accurately as possible the nature of the aberrations in normal physiology which may underlie the phenomenon. It is by no means certain that Raynaud's is a single disorder with a single pathology – there is no reason why several similar entities could not be concealed under this one heading. Careful sifting of clinical data is a very worthwhile exercise; screening for the causes of secondary Raynaud's is certainly essential in any patients being investigated and studies on sufficiently large numbers of patients to accrue data on the exact way in which they respond to cold challenge need to be undertaken to let us understand the problem better. Laboratory investigations are always interesting but care must also be taken to avoid attributing epi-phenomena to part of the disease process itself. It is reasonably obvious that if circulatory standstill occurs in digits or in a limb; changes in clotting factors, be they platelet or endothelially produced, or tissue factors due to deoxygenation and changes in red cells and white cells themselves will certainly take place. Whereas these may be important when one considers the consequences for those who are managed, it is equally important that we distinguish the causes of the symptoms and the results of the event in the first place. This is not always easy as there may be some interplay between the effects and the causes. Complicated – but worth trying to sort out.

As far as the management of Raynaud's is concerned, much valuable work has been done by the Raynaud's Association on the application of everyday practical measures to combat the effects of Raynaud's and the development of simple aids to help people cope with cold weather. The search for medication which will be relatively risk free – nothing is absolutely risk free – continues, with calcium channel antagonists being the most likely candidates at the moment. These certainly do not suit everyone; of course not all individuals are prepared to sustain drug management. The approach of using feedback techniques is one which has been extremely useful in a number of disorders especially when neurologically mediated controls systems are involved. The approach is somewhat time consuming but again for selected patients who are amenable to this kind of treatment these techniques may be ideal.

We are grateful for the support of Bayer UK in the preparation of the book, especially for the coloured illustrations.

Stuart Roath

1 Raynaud's disorder(s) clinical and pathophysiological features

STUART ROATH

In 1862 Maurice Raynaud published a study of 25 patients with peripheral vascular problems. Although the patients themselves probably represented some individuals with primary Raynaud's and others with a variety of Raynaud's associated disorders – secondary Raynaud's – his description of the phenomenon and its subsequent refinement by others particularly by Hutchinson (1901) at the turn of the century and Allan in the early 1930s (Allan and Brown, 1932) have allowed us to make a scientific approach to the understanding, classification and management of the phenomenon.

Typically, Raynaud's phenomenon is associated with exposure to cold although the degree to which it is exhibited is quite variable. Exposure to cold may mean in some individuals anything less than ambient temperature, say the warmest summer's day, whereas other Raynaud's sufferers are only symptomatic when out of doors in the winter and perhaps exposed to not only cold but convection heat loss by wind or evaporated heat loss through wet. I am unaware of any serious attempts to grade Raynaud's by the severity of the stimulus needed to produce the phenomenon nor is it classified by the extensiveness of the phenomenon, despite the recognition by most sufferers and investigators of the disorder that there are these differences. Raynaud's phenomenon may cause problems in up to 5% of the whole population (Porter, 1976). It has also been described in association with emotional stress.

CLINICAL FINDINGS

Characteristically the first symptom is blanching of the fingers or other affected part which may come on without warning. At the same time sensation may be lost and finger or hand movements may become extremely clumsy. Often affected individuals experience difficulty in, for example, cycling, riding, gardening or pegging out clothes. This stage of the Raynaud's 'attack' is followed by cyanosis as the remaining stagnant blood in the finger or whatever tissue is affected becomes deoxygenated; at this point, as is generally true in oxygen-starved tissue, pain may become apparent. The next occurrence in the sequence of events is the return of circulation either due to active warming or relaxation of vasospasm following deoxygenation. This hyperaemic phase is usually accompanied by redness and swelling of the affected area (e.g. digits) and hyperasthesia, sometimes to a very painful degree. There is some variation in the symptoms and some individuals fail to report the blanching: instead they complain of swollen discoloured painful digits only. The fingers, toes or other affected areas vary from one individual to another but in any individual the same digits tend to be most affected. Tissue loss from gangrene or even skin ulcers is uncommon although lesions due to excoriation have been noted. Strictly speaking the term Raynaud's phenomenon should be applied only if the classical triad of pallor, cyanosis and redness occur in sequence. However, many patients will present with a complaint of cold-related pain in the fingers, toes or other sites. Some of these may indeed have primary Raynaud's phenomenon but it is vital that other disorders with symptom presentations mimicking primary Raynaud's be clearly distinguished from the latter as the prognosis and management may be totally different.

OTHER DISORDERS WITH SIMILAR CASE HISTORIES: PRIMARY AND SECONDARY RAYNAUD'S

Symptoms and clinical findings resembling those seen in primary Raynaud's disorder may be found in numerous other conditions. Some of these are vascular disorders in their own right and relatively benign such as acrocyanosis, livedo reticularis or erythromelalgia. Other conditions where such symptoms occur are usually classified as secondary Raynaud's. Some confusion in reports from different sources may be caused by the introduction of terms such as Raynaud's disorder, Raynaud's disease and Raynaud's phenomenon with attempts to apply these to clinical situations where Raynaud's is primary, or secondary to some other disease; but the safest approach is simply to apply the terminology primary Raynaud's when no associated condition is found to cause the symptoms and to use secondary Raynaud's where other disorders with pathology which can

Table 1.1 Disorders exhibiting Raynaud's-like phenomenon (secondary Raynaud's)

1. Connective tissue disorders
    (a) Scleroderma
    (b) CREST Syndrome
    (c) Systemic lupus erythematosus
    (d) Mixed connective tissue disease
    (e) Rheumatoid arthritis
    (f) Dermatomyositis

2. Peripheral vascular disorders
    (a) Arteriosclerosis
    (b) Embolic disease
    (c) Venous thrombosis
    (d) (Thromboangiitis obliterans – diabetes)

3. (Inflammatory) vasculitides

4. Blood abnormalities – protein disorders
                         cellular disorders
                         anaemias

5. Occupational disorders

6. Drug associations

7. Neurological disorders

8. Tumours (Neoplasms)

9. Miscellaneous disorders

lead to Raynaud's-like symptoms can be found. These latter occur in a host of different clinical situations, some of which are listed in Table 1.1 and which will be discussed briefly as follows. Other primary disorders which might be confused with Raynaud's are described afterward.

Connective tissue disorders

Scleroderma and Crest syndrome

Scleroderma and the Crest syndrome (oesophageal hypomotility, sclerodactyly and telangiectasia) are probably the disorders in this group which in the early stages can be identified only as showing Raynaud's phenomenon. Raynaud's may actually precede any noticeable skin changes by months or years and the real diagnosis may not be made until the other manifestations of the disease appear. Fingers and hands are often permanently swollen in the early stages, then in typical cases the skin becomes thickened and atrophic with calcific deposits and breakdown giving painful ulcerative lesions. Sooner or later the facial or other manifestations will also present themselves and about half the patients will also complain of some kind of polyarthritis. Symptoms related to the oesophageal involvement are also present in about half of any series of scleroderma patients and other system manifestations of this multisystem disease such as pulmonary, renal or cardiac involvement will eventually occur. Diagnosis is generally made on clinical grounds but the typical connective disease findings – elevated erythrocyte sedimentation rate, anaemia, increased immunoglobulins, antinuclear antibodies or even rheumatoid factor – may all be found. None of these should be present in patients with primary Raynaud's phenomenon. The Crest syndrome, originally thought to be a limited form of scleroderma, is probably simply a more slowly progressive form of this disease.

The other connective tissue disorders such as systemic lupus erythematosus, mixed connective tissue disease, rheumatoid arthritis or dermatomyositis are probably less often likely to be confused with primary Raynaud's phenomenon and scleroderma with the exception of mixed connective tissue disease where skin over the fingers can be atrophic and telangiectasia may also be present. Biopsy material although perhaps comparable with scleroderma in the skin can also show immunoglobulin deposition in various sites.

Systemic lupus erythematosus

Systemic lupus erythematosus, however, like the former disease, almost invariably shows high antibodies to nucleo protein and because of its frequent association with arthralgia and cutaneous manifestations could be briefly confused with Raynaud's phenomenon. It also occurs in approximately the same sex distribution (1:9 male to female) as Raynaud's phenomenon but because of its multisystem manifestations and variety of laboratory abnormalities the differential diagnosis should not present difficulties. The positive test for antinuclear factor, frequency of anaemia, the hypocomplementaemia and increased gamma globulin are all characteristic of this disorder.

Rheumatoid arthritis

Raynaud's-like phenomena have been reported with this disorder but as there is a considerable cross-over between the manifestations of this problem and the connective tissue diseases it is possible that some of the reports are erroneous or that because both rheumatoid arthritis and Raynaud's are relatively common disorders, especially in women, then some patients with the former will by chance also complain of Raynaud's of a primary type.

Peripheral vascular disorders

Intermittent claudication, embolus or thrombotic arteritis

By far the commonest underlying disorder of these would be arteriosclerosis which frequently manifests itself in its chronic form as coldness of the feet, pain in the feet and especially in the calves if classical intermittent claudication is present. The age and sex incidence, however, is quite different – it is more common in males and relatively uncommon until the fiftieth year of age unless there is some other predisposing disorder. Typically the symptoms, although relieved by warmth or rest are often always present and the abnormal findings in the peripheral or even popliteal pulses are still present when the patient is warm. Examination of the peripheral arterial vasculative which should be normal in primary Raynaud's phenomenon should exclude this differential diagnosis.

Most of the other vascular phenomena, unlike arteriosclerosis, are of a more acute nature. Embolization of a major blood vessel with its accompanying pain and shock should not be diagnostically confused with Raynaud's, but recurrent multiple small emboli with digital symptoms could be possibly viewed as such, especially in an individual who perhaps had atrial fibrillation. It is unlikely that the classical cold-associated phenomena would be described however. Much the same applies to venous thrombosis where the symptoms are largely pain and swelling and not really cold related.

Diabetes

In diabetes the combination of arteriopathy and neuropathy, accompanied by threatened or real tissue loss in the extremities might just be confused with primary Raynaud's. Blood flow studies in diabetics with severe neuropathy can undoubtedly show that they still respond to cold, which would make the vasoconstriction worse. However, diabetics often have deprivation of sensation from their feet with neuropathic ulceration and progressive tissue loss. The combination of arteriopathy and neuropathy seen in some degree in about half the patients with advanced diabetes and its progressive nature should not present difficulties in distinction from primary Raynaud's.

Vasculitis

Vasculitis – most commonly arteritis – has as its pathogenesis inflammatory lesions of the blood vessel walls. There is a variety of disorders seen under this heading. The nomenclature is determined usually by the site of the pathology or by the symptom complex associated with the disorder. Briefly the vasculitides may be classified as:

1. hypersensitivity associated
2. allergic
3. rheumatic

4. periarteritis nodosa
5. temporal arteritis

They are often described as necrotizing vasculitides or angiitides. For the present purposes many of them are unlikely ever to be confused with Raynaud's but among the hypersensitivity-associated disorders, Henoch–Schoenlein purpura may have involvement of the digits, tip of the nose or ears. The clinical situation however, is quite well defined – it is normally a disorder of childhood, an acute febrile illness characterized by fever, joint pains, abdominal pain and often renal failure. The characteristic purpura should not be confused with cold-associated colour changes of true Raynaud's.

Other vasculitic disorders include the vasculitis of rheumatoid arthritis and systemic lupus erythematosus which has already been discussed. Disorders such as Wegener's granulomatosis and allergic granulomatous angiites, polyarteritis nodosa may, among their multisystem clinical manifestations, occasionally present with digital ischaemia and even gangrene. As they are a somewhat more insidious disorder than acute vasculitides and may present in later life, they might just possibly be considered in an older individual who presents with digital problems which may mimic Raynaud's.

In none of the disorders mentioned are there significant cold-associated changes, although exposure to cold could obviously worsen symptoms if those of peripheral vascular impairment were already present. Purpura, tissue loss and systemic illnesses are the characteristics of the vasculitic group of disorders – features not found in primary Raynaud's.

Blood abnormalities

Paraproteinaemias

Individuals with pathologically high levels of circulating immunoglobulins – usually monoclonal – such as in myeloma or macroglobulinaemia – may show Raynaud's like phenomena especially when these proteins are cold precipitable as they are in cryoglobulinaemias. Examination of the blood will often show spontaneous agglutination or rouleaux formation. The age of onset is usually older than that of Raynaud's but there is some overlap in the presentation and symptomatology so careful history taking and screening may be necessary to identify these disorders. As the management is totally different from that of primary Raynaud's this of course is most important.

Cryoglobulinaemia

Although many cryoglobulins are associated with the malignant paraproteinaemias there is another group – essential mixed cryoglobulinaemia – which appears to be distinct from these disorders. Raynaud's phenomenon is certainly complained of especially in the early stages of this disorder and it usually progresses fairly rapidly with arthralgia, purpura and haematuria. In this respect it begins to resemble vasculitis and therefore occupies an intermediate position between the paraproteinaemias and the vasculitides. It can appear at any age and affect either sex and, like many of the rheumatoid disorders, exhibit a high erythrocyte sedimentation rate which would be unexpected in primary Raynaud's and cause gross precipitation in the blood – a gel often being formed – which again is not a finding in primary Raynaud's.

Cold agglutinins or cold haemagglutinins

An important differential from primary Raynaud's is a group of disorders where exposure to cold precipitates red blood cell agglutination. As in the previous group of paraproteinaemias, blood viscosity is increased in this situation and peripheral circulation may be moderately or even grossly impaired. This cold-induced disorder may be associated with red blood cell destruction due to complement activation linked with this phenomenon. This is probably the same phenomenon as cold haemolysis and may be accompanied by haemoglobinuria. Elevated and clinically significant cold agglutinin titres are often secondary to lymphoproliferative or myeloproliferative disorders and occasionally to collagen disorders or infectious agents such as mycoplasma. In some individuals, however, the disease does seem idiopathic. This disorder is one of the most important to distinguish from primary Raynaud's. The age/sex presentation is unhelpful – it has been reported at all ages – but careful history taking should show that the digits are more generally involved and that there is no phase of vasoconstriction as in primary Raynaud's. Many patients with cold agglutinins will of course have evidence of their primary disorder, e.g. some will be anaemic.

Cold agglutinins, however, are often found in individuals who are otherwise perfectly normal and it can be difficult to decide in a given patient with Raynaud's phenomenon who also has circulating cold agglutinins whether in fact the latter are the important pathobiological factors in causation of the phenomenon. Generally speaking low-titre cold agglutinins (e.g. up to 1:64) may well be irrelevant and cold agglutinins of restricted thermal amplitude, e.g. below 18°C, may also be of less importance. However, it can sometimes be impossible to rule out cold agglutinins as being responsible for the individual's problems in Raynaud's when both they and primary Raynaud's are present.

Cryofibrinoginaemia, sometimes in association with chronic disseminated intravascular coagulation, can sometimes be seen as a rather severe acute form of secondary Raynaud's phenomenon and because of deposition of fibrin in small arterioles it may be associated with digital thrombosis and tissue loss.

Anaemia is a fairly common problem affecting women in the same range span as primary Raynaud's. In younger patients more obvious symptoms such as dyspnoea on exertion may be ignored and generalized complaints such as lassitude and coldness in the hands and fingers may occasionally be confused with Raynaud's.

Thrombocythaemia

In this disorder and in some cases of polycythaemia with high platelet counts ($>700 \times 10^9$/l) sludging of platelet aggregates may occur in the peripheral circulation with complaints of coldness, discolouration, ulceration, tissue loss and sometimes loss of digits or even limbs. This is usually a severe problem occurring in somewhat older patients who present with apparent Raynaud's and its early recognition (and treatment) is essential to prevent continued tissue loss. The classical triad of symptoms of primary Raynaud's is not present and there is no relief of symptoms on warming.

Occupational disorders associated with Raynaud's phenomenon

Vibration white finger (occupational vibration disease)

Raynaud's syndrome or a strikingly similar disorder is seen in individuals using, for example, pneumatic drills, chainsaws or grinding or polishing wheels. Its prevalence is said to be up to 90% in some studies of chainsaw operators and grinders and up to 50% in pneumatic drillers. The changes seem to be confined to digits of the appropriate hand or hands only and are presumably mediated through local vascular reflex arcs. No evidence exists to suggest that these individuals are especially predisposed to Raynaud's (no family history, usually males and no signs of the disease elsewhere), but there are most certainly pathophysiological factors in common and there are reports of success with the same kinds of drugs as are used in primary Raynaud's phenomenon.

Trauma

Direct trauma to the arteries is also recorded as giving problems with peripheral circulation – the hypothenar-hammer syndrome which damages the ulnar artery is an example of this disorder but there is no reason why this should be aetiologically confused with Raynaud's phenomenon.

Chemical exposure induced Raynaud's phenomenon

One of the best known historically has been that disorder occurring in workers exposed to vinyl chloride. This is sometimes called occupational acro-osteolysis which clinically may resemble scleroderma and indeed may have a similar pathogenesis. X-rays of the hands in this disorder will reveal the characteristic changes in the terminal phalanges and, as a preventable disease, it should not be seen nowadays.

Drug-associated Raynaud's phenomenon

More importantly Raynaud's phenomenon may be seen as a side effect of drug treatment in a number of disorders. Historically perhaps the best known is ergot.

Ergot

This drug is still used in the treatment of migraine and of course it is present in nature as a fungal infestation of rye. The vasospasm caused by ergot, however, may be sustained and lead to digital gangrene as opposed to the intermittent nature of primary Raynaud's and the rarity of tissue loss in that disorder.

Other drugs of this kind, e.g. boromocriptine and methysergide, are also capable of producing Raynaud's phenomenon. All these drugs are currently in use.

Beta-blocking drugs

Beta adrenergic blocking drugs, of which propranolol is probably the best known, give rise to Raynaud's phenomenon as an occasional side effect. The incidence is variable although up to 50% have been reported. Most cases must be mild and probably subclinical although tissue loss has actually been reported in this situation. The pathogenesis of this particular disorder is probably associated with a fall in digital arterial blood pressure and an inability to respond correctly to cooling. Perhaps alpha-receptor sensitivity enhancement may occur in the presence of beta-receptor blockade.

Cytotoxic agents

An increasing number of cases with Raynaud's phenomenon have been described in patients given bleomycin either alone or with other agents particularly vincristine. Its association occasionally with platinum in some modern chemotherapeutic programmes may be interesting, as heavy metals (historically lead and arsenic) have also been associated with peripheral vascular problems. The effects are likely to be direct ones on the musculature of the blood vessels – a phenomenon which is not seen in primary Raynaud's disorder.

Contraceptive pills

A variety of Raynaud-like effects have been reported with contraceptive pills or the cessation of this treatment. Despite an early report of severe digital ischaemia with tissue loss, this must be an extremely rare phenomenon and as it is not reported in a recent epidemiological study which included the effects of the pill on improvement or otherwise of Raynaud's. Probably it is not a significant finding.

Miscellaneous conditions

There are a number of apparent unrelated clinical situations where Raynaud's phenomenon or symptom complexes resembling this are reported.

Post-traumatic reflex sympathetic dystrophy

This is a well-reported disorder following injury or operation on a limb. The leg seems to be the commonest site but it is also seen following operations or damage to the arm. The affected limb shows swelling, discolouration with peripheral vasodilatation and cold sensitivity but occasionally pallor or cold-associated pain resembling Raynaud's may be complained of. If this is associated with peripheral nerve injury persistent burning pain (causalgia) may be experienced.

Neurological disorders associated with Raynaud's

There are some fairly obvious compression syndromes which may be associated with Raynaud's especially in the hands. These include the thoracic outlet syndrome, crutch pressure in the axilla and the carpaltunnel syndrome. In all these situations a mixture of nerve and vascular compression may well be the pathogenesis of the complaint of pain, which may be worsened by cold, colour changes due to direct vascular compression or aberrant neurological control of the blood vessels. These changes, however, would rarely be bilateral and the classical sequence of events in primary Raynaud's phenomenon would not be seen.

Occasionally complaints of pain, coldness or discolouration in limbs following hemiplegia are noted but again it is unlikely that these will be confused with primary Raynaud's syndrome.

Neoplasms

Rarely digital ischaemia seems to have been associated with occult neoplasia in the absence of any links such as cryoglobulins or paraproteinaemia although some of the older reports undoubtedly included well-defined secondary Raynaud's.

Chronic renal failure

A few reports of arterial calcinosis and peripheral tissue-loss associated with chronic renal failure have been reported. Again the persistence of the problem and a difficulty to relieve with warming – typical of any disorder where there is actual damage to the peripheral blood vessels – should make it easy to distinguish from primary Raynaud's disorder.

Hypothyroidism

Historically hypothyroidism has been regarded as a treatable cause of Raynaud's phenomenon. It has been reported both in primary and secondary hypothyroidism and is presumably associated with an increased sensitivity to adrenergic stimulation which has been noted in experimental studies of this disorder.

Other cold-associated disorders

Chilblains, prurigo and cold urticaria. Although it is unlikely that any of these would be confused with primary Raynaud's phenomenon they should perhaps be recorded. Chilblains are relatively common in children whereas true Raynaud's is rare in this group, although there are some reports of severe cases in childhood. Prurigo and cold urticaria are historically different and not to be confused with primary Raynaud's.

Other primary Raynaud-like disorders (Table 1.2)

Acrocyanosis

In this rare disorder which occurs most commonly in young women, there is a distant diffuse cyanosis and coldness of the fingers and toes and sometimes of the hands and feet. It is usually present during both warm and cold weather although the disorder tends to persist during warm weather. The complaint is one of coldness rather than variable colour or abnormalities of sensation. It is a benign disorder and it is not associated with ulceration or progression to, for example, a collagen disorder.

Table 1.2   Other primary disorders of the vascular response

Acrocyanosis
Livedo reticularis
Erythromelalgia
Chilblains ⎫
Prurigo   ⎬ Cold associated
Urticaria ⎭

Livedo reticularis

Again this is usually, although not invariably, a benign disorder with a bluish mottled appearance of the skin most commonly over the lower legs. The idiopathic form which is usual is more or less permanent and detectable even in warm weather. A variant may be more sensitive to temperature. Usually there are no associated problems but in occasional cases vague symptoms of discomfort may occur. A small number of cases are said to be associated with underlying collagen or vascular disorders and occasionally tissue loss may occur. The benign form is, however, far more common.

Erythromelalgia

This should not be confused with Raynaud's disease as the symptoms tend to appear on warming when hyperaesthesia and itching of the hands or lower legs occurs. The skin is often warm and red or reddish-blue. Skin lesions do not result although sometimes the itching is so severe that excoriation may occur from scratching. It is not associated with any group of underlying disorders.

It is difficult to tell what percentage of patients presenting with Raynaud's phenomenon will have primary or secondary Raynaud's. Figure 1.1 (reproduced by permission of the Arthritis Foundation) suggests that about three quarters of all Raynaud's will be primary. It is, therefore, important that the substantial minority of patients with secondary Raynaud's have a correct

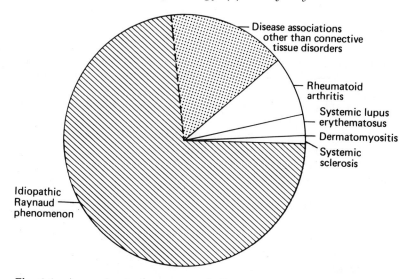

Fig. 1.1 Approximate frequency of disease associations with new cases of Raynaud's phenomenon (see text)

diagnosis assigned because frequently the Raynaud's phenomenon will be associated with the critical need for appropriate management of the underlying disorder. Treating the Raynaud's phenomenon itself would be of little benefit to a patient who, for example, has cold agglutinin disease or one of the connective tissue disorders. A guide to the assessment of patients presenting apparently with Raynaud's phenomenon is shown in Table 1.3.

THE PATHOLOGY OF PRIMARY RAYNAUD'S

The blood flow to the digits is extremely variable and may be unrecordable in normal individuals during severe vasoconstriction. This is a perfectly normal phenomenon. In severe cold, (low temperatures, 0–10°C), vasoconstriction is interrupted by temporary vasodilation, a mechanism probably designed to prevent skin necrosis, whereas at slightly higher temperatures vasoconstriction can be longer lasting.

The mechanism of vasoconstriction is accepted as being through sympathetic stimulation of alpha-adrenergic receptors

Table 1.3 An approach to the diagnosis of Raynaud's phenomenon

---

History
1. Elicit classical triad of peripheral colour changes and associated timing of symptoms
   Check persistence of symptoms during warming
   Relation of symptoms to exercise or stress

2. Family history

3. Review of other systems to rule out secondary Raynaud's general symptoms
   weight loss
   weakness
   fever
   arthritis
   skin rashes

4. Social history and occupational background
   Smoking history
   Relationship of symptoms to pregnancies, menarche or menopause

5. Drug history

6. History of trauma or previous surgery

Physical examination
If possible observe the sequence of colour change and the accompanying effect
Note skin or tissue loss or ulceration
Skin colour, rashes or purpura
Joint abnormalities
Arterial pulses
Adenopathy, organomegaly, signs of anaemia, general condition

Laboratory investigations
Full blood count, haemoglobin, platelets, WBC ESR or equivalent
Autoimmune profile with special reference to anti-nuclear factor and rheumatoid factor
Fibrinogen and assessment of fibrinogenic state
Examination for cold-associated proteins and immunoglobin levels

---

in the small arterioles – vasodilation is presumably a passive relaxation following such stimulation. (Although the beta-adrenergic receptors may also cause stimulation and vasodilation.) These mechanisms are also generally responsible for the maintenance of blood pressure, although other arteries and arterioles are involved in addition. Patients with Raynaud's phenomenon tend to be hypersensitive to vasomotor stimuli – they are said to have 'Raynaud's like' changes in response to emotional stress and even at normal temperatures seem to show more tendency to skin colouration and sweating. Tests of vasomotor function and variability in the contents of the blood vessels have been exhaustively undertaken in Raynaud's and some of the results are presented in later chapters. So far no clear, single pathological defect has been found in primary Raynaud's. This may be because the vasomotor changes are only slightly altered from the normal or that there may be several different mechanisms involved even in primary Raynaud's causing a lack of uniformity in reported data on the pathology of the problem.

There are two approaches to Raynaud's. One would suggest the findings are part of a spectrum of normal responses to cold – the 'top end' of the response curve as it were; the other approach is to consider Raynaud's as a 'disease' where the response is definitely pathological. The other interesting concept is that of the linkage between Raynaud's, industrial vibration white finger and cold injury, e.g. frost bite, frost nip, or immersion injury. It seems likely that many common phenomena will be observed in these defined clinical situations, true primary Raynaud's – assuming this exists – and normal individuals who suffer from cold. What needs to be carefully distinguished are the many epiphenomena described which occur as a result of cold sensitivity or cold itself, and any underlying data which reveal disease pathogenesis. The former will probably include changes in endothelial and platelet activation, and their products; possible changes in red cell deformability due to deoxygenation and changes in whole blood viscosity, again associated with cold, stasis, and changes in pH. The latter type of changes – those basic to Raynaud's – are more likely to include dynamic alterations in vasomotor responses, numbers of neural receptors or increased sensitivity to vasoconstrictive messages.

Currently the most important diagnostic aspect of Raynaud's

is to ensure that those cases of secondary Raynaud's are correctly identified and that in the search for pathogenic mechanisms they are distinguished from primary disorders, also that epiphenomena reasonably expected to follow vasoconstriction or cold exposure should not be mistaken for the fundamental pathophysiology of Raynaud's.

REFERENCES

Allan, E.V. and Brown, G.E. (1932) Raynaud's Disease. A clinical study of one hundred and forty seven cases. *J. Am. Med. Assoc.* **99**, 1472.
Hutchinson, J. (1901) Raynaud's phenomenon. *Med. Press Cir.*, **123**, 403–5.
Porter, J.M. (1976) The clinical significance of Raynaud's syndrome. *Surgery*, **80**, 756–64.

FURTHER READING

Blunt, R.J. and Poster, J.M. (1986) Raynaud's syndrome. *Semin. Arth. Rheum.*, **10**, 282.
Friedman, S.A. (ed.) (1982) *Abnormalities of vasomotor tone in vascular disease.* J. Wright, Boston, pp. 43–86.
McGarth, M.A. and Penny, R. (1974) The mechanisms of Raynaud's phenomenon (Res 1 + 2). *Med. J. Aust.* **2**, 328–33 and 367–75.
Nilsen, K.H. (1980) Pathophysiological classification of Raynaud's phenomenon. *Br. J. Dermatol.*, **102**, 1–5.
Raynaud, M. (1888) On asphyxia and symmetrical gangrene of the extremities, and new researches on the nature and treatment of local asphyxia of the extremities. (Translated by Thomas Barlow), New Sydenham Society, London.

2 The epidemiology of Raynaud's phenomenon

VIVIAN CHALLENOR

Maurice Raynaud in his thesis of 1862 first described a phenomenon characterized by symmetrical intermittent reversible vasospasm of the arteries, which has subsequently come to bear his name. One major difficulty in obtaining accurate epidemiological data has been the heterogeneous nature of Raynaud's phenomenon. Rigid application of Raynaud's original diagnostic criteria requires the occurrence of all three phases of a classical attack. It has now become apparent that many patients with Raynaud's phenomenon do not describe classical attacks, or at least, all the features of such an attack. Following Raynaud's initial description, both Hutchinson (1901) and Allen and Brown (1932) modified diagnostic criteria in an attempt to improve patient identification. In general, variations on these criteria have been used to identify patients in epidemiologal surveys.

PREVALENCE OF RAYNAUD'S PHENOMENON

Surprisingly few studies have assessed the prevalence of Raynaud's phenomenon in the general population (Table 2.1). Estimates of prevalence range from 0.06 to 30% in different population samples. A number of factors account for the wide variation in these results from population studies. First, the populations sampled differed in terms of their country and often continent of origin, ethnic complement and sex distribution. Second, study designs have varied markedly. In particular those based on questionnaires have resulted in the inclusion of patients with cold sensitivity who do not fulfil accepted diagnostic criteria for Raynaud's phenomenon.

Maricq *et al*. (1986) in a study (underaken in South Carolina) of 1752 randomly selected subjects, described on overall preva-

Table 2.1 The prevalence of Raynaud's phenomenon in the general population

Source	%	
Lewis (1929)	27	
NHANES (1974)	0.83	
Fessel (1975)	14	
Olsen and Nielsen (1978)	22	(young female, only)
Heslop et al. (1983)	13	
Maricq et al. (1986)	1.9	(10% prevalence of cold sensitivity)
Leppert et al. (1987)	15.6	(female only)

lence of 'cold sensitivity' of approximately 10%. The study was based on a short questionnaire. When specific criteria for the diagnosis of Raynaud's phenomenon such as cold sensitivity with digital colour changes and cold sensitivity leading to medical consultation were combined, overall prevalence was reduced to 1.9%. This value was considerably lower than most of the previous studies. Although there is little evidence to suggest that a cold climate is an aetiological factor of Raynaud's phenomenon, it is conceivable that a significant number of Maricq's patients with cold sensitivity did not exhibit digital colour changes due to the relative warmth of the climate in South Carolina.

This view would be supported by the study by Heslop, Coggan and Acheson (1983) who looked at a general practice sample of subjects in Southampton, UK. An overall prevalence of 13% of Raynaud's phenomenon was described, following correction for false positives in the sample using the diagnostic criteria laid down by Allen and Brown (1932).

The study by Fessel (1975) showed comparable results with a prevalence of 14% using slightly different diagnostic criteria. Olsen and Nielson (1978) studied Swedish female physical therapists only and found a prevalence of 22%. Since the prevalence of Raynaud's phenomenon is higher in females (subsequently discussed) their higher reported values are not unexpected.

A recent study by Leppert et al. (1987) assessed the prevalence of Raynaud's phenomenon in a random sample of 2705 Swedish women aged 18–59 years: 19% complained of cold white fingers with or without numbness. Following interview and examination 79% were believed to have Raynaud's phenomenon resulting in an overall prevalence of 15.6%. However, once again only females were studied. One study, the National Health and Nutrition Examination Survey (1974), reported an extremely low prevalence of Raynaud's phenomenon. However, this was based on unknown diagnostic criteria during a single dermatological examination. It is likely that a gross underestimation of prevalence occurred.

In summary it is likely that the overall prevalence rate of Raynaud's phenomenon in the general population lies between 10 and 15% depending on the diagnostic criteria used and the population (and its environment) studied.

By its very nature the relative frequency of primary and secondary Raynaud's phenomenon can only be adequately assessed in the hospital setting. The results of a number of studies over the last 30 years are shown (Table 2.2). Interestingly there appeared to be an apparent increase in the prevalence of secondary Raynaud's phenomenon from 1956 (23%) to 1976 (94%) in patients attending hospital. However, this may be explained purely on the grounds of improved diagnostic facilities over the last 30 years. The use of sophisticated immunological techniques had identified not only patients with autoimmune disease, but also patients with immunological abnormalities without severe clinical symptoms. It is mainly the inclusion of the latter group that has led to the apparent reverse in the relative prevalence of primary and secondary Raynaud's phenomenon. The most recent and comprehensive study was under-

Table 2.2 Relative prevalence of primary and secondary Raynaud's phenomenon among patients attending hospital clinics

Reference	No of patients	Primary Raynaud's	Secondary Raynaud's
Blain *et al.* (1951)	238	119 (50%)	119 (50%)
Gifford and Hines (1957)	629	464 (77%)	165 (23%)
Velayos *et al.* (1971)	137	28 (20%)	109 (80%)
Sumner and Strandness (1972)	105	16 (15%)	89 (85%)
Porter *et al.* (1976)	100	19 (19%)	81 (81%)

taken by Porter *et al.* (1976) who studied a consecutive group of 100 patients presenting with Raynaud's symptoms. Clinical and immunological evaluation resulted in the following diagnosis: 28 with scleroderma or CREST, 10 with systemic lupus erythematosus (SLE), 43 with miscellaneous autoimmune disease. A total of 19 had no diagnosable autoimmune disease although 14 had serological abnormalities. Therefore, the overall prevalence of primary Raynaud's phenomenon in this group was 5% of patients with Raynaud's syndrome.

However, this merely describes patients with symptoms severe enough to warrant a hospital consultation. It is likely that many patients experience mild symptoms and do not warrant such specialized consultation. Therefore, it is unlikely that these results bear any relationship to the true prevalence of primary Raynaud's phenomenon as a percentage of all patients with Raynaud's phenomenon in the general population. Although sophisticated diagnostic techniques may discover many more patients with serological disorders it remains likely that the majority of patients in the general population will have primary Raynaud's phenomenon.

SEX RATIOS IN RAYNAUD'S PHENOMENON

Raynaud's phenomenon, particularly when primary, is usually seen in young women. Of Raynaud's original subjects 20 were

Table 2.3 Sex ratios in Raynaud's phenomenon

Source	Females (%)	Males (%)	Sex ratio F:M
General population			
Lewis (1929)	30	25	1.2:1
Fessel (1975)	17	11	1.6:1
Olsen and Nielson (1978)	22	–	–
Heslop *et al.* (1983)	17	8	2.1:1
Maricq *et al.* (1986)			1.3:1
Hospital clinics			
Hines and Christensen (1945)	23	77	3.4:1
Allen and Brown (1932)	76	24	7.8:1
Porter *et al.* (1976)			3.2:1

women (Raynaud, 1888). The greater prevalence of this condition in women has been noted on a number of occasions (Monro, 1899; Spittel, 1972). Reports from the literature suggest a male : female ratio of between 1 : 10 and 1 : 15. This, however, is not borne out by close examination of the major studies undertaken on Raynaud's phenomenon over the last 50 years (Table 2.3). Studies in the general population have suggested male : female ratios of between 1 : 1.2 and 1 : 2.1. Heslop, Coggan and Acheson (1983) found a male : female prevalence of 1 : 2.1 when examining equal numbers of males and females.

One possibility is that previous values were obtained from patients attending hospital clinics. In general, women are more likely to experience autoimmune disorders, e.g. SLE, scleroderma, rheumatoid arthritis, and this may bias the overall results. However, when the results of studies carried out on hospital patients are examined (Table 2.3) the maximum male : female ratio was 1 : 7.8.

Furthermore in the study of Porter *et al.* (1976), the male : female ratio of patients eventually diagnosed as having primary Raynaud's phenomenon was approximately 1 : 1.

It appears likely that previous authors have overestimated the relative numbers of women compared to men who experience Raynaud's phenomenon.

AGE

Most authors agree that the greatest incidence of onset of Raynaud's phenomenon is below the fourth decade. Allen and Brown (1932) found that 73% of patients developed Raynaud's phenomenon before 40 years, with an age range of 5 to 53. Gifford and Hines (1957) found a mean age of 31 years in 474 female patients; 78% were below 39 years with an age range of 4 to 68 years. Heslop, Coggan and Acheson (1983) in a study of equal numbers of males and females in the general population aged between 20 and 59 years, found that 78% experienced the onset of symptoms before 35 years.

Although Raynaud's phenomenon has been reported in a 5-month-old infant (Sayre, 1973) it is a rare condition in children. When it does occur, it is often in connection with connective tissue disorders. Emery and Schaller (1977) in a report of nine children with Raynaud's phenomenon found that five had scleroderma, two had mixed connective tissue disease and one had systemic lupus erythematosus. Again, however, this was a highly specialized group of children attending a hospital clinic.

RACE AND CLIMATE

Maricq *et al*. (1986) reported a similar prevalence of cold sensitivity amongst blacks and whites (22% and 19% respectively). However, although the prevalence was roughly equivalent amongst black and white females, black males showed a slightly higher prevalence (12%) than white males (8%).

There is no evidence that a cold climate is an aetiological factor of Raynaud's phenomenon. Indeed more false positives may have been included in studies undertaken in cold countries.

FAMILY HISTORY

Few studies have examined the prevalence of symptoms amongst first-degree relatives of patients with Raynaud's phenomenon. The studies that do exist suggest cold sensitivity is more common among female relatives. Maricq *et al*. (1986) reported cold sensitivity in 12% of mothers and 5% of sisters of patients with Raynaud's, although a similar prevalence was found in relatives of the control group. Gifford and Hines (1957) found symptoms in 20 family members out of 474 female patients; the majority of the relatives being female.

HORMONAL INFLUENCES

Raynaud's phenomenon appears to be more prevalent among young women, although no satisfactory explanation has been suggested to account for this sex difference. In addition a remission of symptoms has often been noted during pregnancy. In view of their findings a number of authors have suggested that hormonal influences may play a part. Lafferty *et al*. (1985) assessed the effect of cyclic sex hormone fluctuations on the digital vascular reactivity of ten normal young women. The latter was assessed by means of thermal entrainment of finger blood flow and Doppler ultrasound mapping of the digital arteries. In the pre-ovulatory period significant reduction in digital vascular flow was noted. Nine out of ten women had thermal entrainment results similar to those seen in patients with established Raynaud's phenomenon. Furthermore, the fluctuation normally seen in digital vascular flow became less frequent as the subject approached the day of ovulation. Oestrogen is prone to increase the sensitivity of small arteries to adrenaline and noradrenaline (Altura, 1975). This effect may be prevented by the concurrent administration of progesterone. The latter also promotes calcium uptake by smooth muscle endoplasmic reticulum (Carsten, 1979) which inhibits vascular smooth muscle contraction.

Lafferty *et al*. (1985) suggested that primary Raynaud's phenomenon commonly seen in young women is caused by 'an exaggerated vascular response to normal (or possibly abnormal) fluctuations in female sex hormones'. Furthermore, the improvement in symptoms noted during pregnancy could be related to the alteration in the progresterone/oestrogen ratio.

Perhaps not surprisingly in view of the above findings, anecdotal evidence suggests an increased incidence of Raynaud's phenomenon in females taking the pill. The contraceptive pill increases fibrinogen levels in addition to influencing vascular reactivity and subsequently whole blood viscosity. This has been postulated as a possible pathogenetic mechanism in Raynaud's phenomenon.

Jarret (1976) described three patients with Raynaud's phenomenon, who, on stopping the contraceptive pill, were noted to have a decrease in fibrinogen levels and an improvement in symptoms. One of the three patients took a progesterone-only pill, with again a decrease in fibrinogen levels and an improvement in symptoms. He concluded that the contraceptive pill was contraindicated in patients with primary Raynaud's phenomenon or when secondary to scleroderma.

Eastcott (1976) reported the development of Raynaud's phenomenon in three patients, two of whom had diabetes and one scleroderma, on commencing the contraceptive pill. Symptoms disappeared on stopping the pill.

Although little hard scientific evidence exists to support these anecdotal reports, it would appear prudent to employ high oestrogen-containing oral contraceptives with care in patients with Raynaud's phenomenon, particularly in view of the influence of oestrogen on vascular reactivity described by Lafferty *et al*. (1985).

SMOKING

Similar anecdotal evidence exists with respect to an increased incidence of Raynaud's phenomenon among smokers. Bocanegra and Espinoza (1980) described a case in which passive inhalation of nicotine appeared to produce the symptoms of Raynaud's phenomenon. A 47-year-old female presented with a nine-month history of Raynaud's phenomenon. Although a non-smoker, her husband to whom she had been married for 2.5 years smoked 4.5 packets of cigarettes per day. Interestingly the husband had mild Raynaud's phenomenon. Furthermore, he had previously been married to a 48-year-old woman who developed Raynaud's phenomenon on exposure to cold during the last few years of their marriage. When the husband smoked in a separate room, the second wife's symptoms disappeared completely. Passive inhalation of nicotine has been shown to reduce instantaneous blood flow and increase vascular resistance (Coffman, 1967). It is therefore, perhaps, not surprising that Raynaud's phenomenon could be induced in this way.

By contrast Leppert *et al.* (1987) did not find a higher percentage of smokers among patients with Raynaud's phenomenon than among those without. Certainly direct evidence linking smoking to the development of Raynaud's phenomenon is somewhat lacking.

However, smoking may result in an incidence of atheroma leading to secondary Raynaud's phenomenon. Buerger's disease (thromboangiitis obliterans) may lead to Raynaud's phenomenon. Although its cause is unknown it is related to a heavy smoking history. Again, nicotine is known to induce vascular spasms – the basic underlying disorder in Raynaud's phenomenon. It would therefore appear, on the limited evidence available, that patients with Raynaud's phenomenon should avoid smoking.

ASSOCIATION WITH THE OTHER VASOSPASTIC DISORDERS

Since the underlying pathophysiological mechanism involved in the production of an attack of Raynaud's phenomenon is vasospasm, it is not surprising that an increased incidence of the former has been noted in the conditions associated with vascular spasm. A number of authors have commented on the association between migraine and Raynaud's phenomenon (Levy, 1983). Atkinson and Appenzeller (1976) suggested that migraine and Raynaud's phenomenon were merely different manifestations of the same disease.

Miller *et al.* (1981) described an increased incidence of both Raynaud's phenomenon and migraine in patients with variant angina. The authors suggested that variant angina was merely the coronary manifestation of a generalized vasospastic disorder. Similar conclusions were reached by Zahavi *et al.* (1984).

By contrast Leppert *et al.* (1987) reported that although recurrent chest pain and headache were reported significantly more often in patients with Raynaud's phenomenon compared to controls, there was also a higher frequency of recurrent chest pain and headache in a group of patients with non-specific numbness of the fingers than in controls. Furthermore, only a few patients with Raynaud's phenomenon had coronary artery disease, and this number did not differ from that in a control group. He suggested a possible cause of the chest pain might be a disordered muscle microcirculation as described in primary fibromyalgia (Bengtsson, 1986), or possibly because Raynaud's patients are more polysymptomatic.

In conclusion it would appear that some individuals do develop a generalized vasospastic disorder the manifestation and severity of which differ widely. This may explain the increased incidence of chest pain in some but not all patients with Raynaud's phenomenon. Raynaud's phenomenon would, therefore, appear to be at one end of a spectrum of disorders, the pathogenesis (and treatment) of which remains unsatisfactory.

REFERENCES

Allen, E.V. and Brown, G.E. (1932) Raynaud's disease: A critical review of minimal requisites for diagnosis. *Am. J. Med. Sci.*, **183**, 187.

Altura, B.M. (1975) Sex and oestrogen and responsiveness of terminal arterioles to neurohypophysial hormones and catecholamines. *J. Pharm. Exp. Ther.*, **193**, 403–12.

Atkinson, A.R. and Appenzeller, O. (1976) Hemicrania and Raynaud's phenomenon: Manifestation of the same disease? *Headache*, **16**, 1–2.

Bengtsson, A. (1986) Primary fibromyalgia: A clinical and laboratory study. Linkoping University Medical Dissertations No. 224, Linkoping.

Blain, A. III., Coller, F.A. and Carver, G.B. (1951) Raynaud's disease: A study of criteria for prognosis. *Surgery*, **29**, 387–97.

Bocanegra, T.S. and Espinoza, L.R. (1980) Raynaud's phenomenon in passive smokers. *N. Engl. J. Med.*, **303**, 1419.

Carsten, M.E. (1979) Calcium accumulation by human uterine microsomal preparations: effects of progesterone and oxytocin. *Am. J. Obstet. Gynecol.*, **133**, 598–601.

Coffman, J.D. (1967) The attenuation by reserpine or guanethidine of the cutaneous vasoconstriction caused by tobacco smoke. *Am. Heart J.*, **74**, 229–34.

Eastcott, H.H. (1976) Raynaud's disease and the oral contraceptive pill. *Br. Med. J.*, **2**, 477.

Emery, H. and Schaller, J. (1977) Raynaud's phenomenon in childhood. *Arthr. Rheum.*, (Suppl.) **20**, 363.

Fessel, W.J. (1975) Rheumatology for clinicians. Stratton, New York, p. 214.

Gifford, R.W. and Hines, E.A. (1957) Raynaud's disease among women and girls. *Circulation*, 1012–21.

Heslop, J., Coggan, D. and Acheson, E.D. (1983) The prevalence of intermittent digital ischaemia (Raynaud's phenomenon) in a general practice. *J. Royal Coll. Gen. Pract.*, **33**, 85–9.

Hines, E.A. and Christensen, N.A. (1945) Raynaud's disease among men. *J. Am. Med. Assoc.*, **129**, 1.

Hutchinson, J. (1901) Raynaud's phenomenon. *Med. Press*, **72**, 403.

Jarret, P. E. (1976) Raynaud's disease and oral contraceptives. *Br. Med. J.*, **2**, 699.

Lafferty, K., De Trafford, J.C., Potter, C., Roberts, V.C. and Cotton, L.T. (1985) Reflex vascular responses in the finger to contralateral thermal stimuli during the normal menstrual cycle: a hormonal basis to Raynaud's phenomenon? *Clin. Sci.*, **68**, 639–45.

Leppert, J., Aberg, H., Ringovist, I. and Sorensson, S. (1987) Prevalence of Raynaud's phenomenon in the general population. *Angiology*, **38**, 871–7.

Levy, L.M. (1983) An epidemiological study of headache in an urban population in Zimbabwe. *Headache*, **23**, 2–9.

Lewis, T. (1929) Experiments relating to the peripheral mechanism involved in spasmodic arrest of the circulation in the fingers, a variety of Raynaud's disease. *Heart*, **15**, 7–101.

Maricq, H.R., Weinrich, M.C., Keil, J.E. and Leroy, E.C. (1986) Prevalence of Raynaud's phenomenon in the general population. *J. Chron. Dis.*, **39**, 423–7.

Miller, D., Waters, D.D., Warnica, W., Szlachcic, J., Kreeft, J. and Theroux, P. (1981) Is variant angina the coronary manifestation of a generalised vasospastic disorder? *N. Engl. J. Med.*, **304**, 763–6.

Monro, T.K. (1899) *Raynaud's Disease*. James Maclehose, Glasgow.

Olsen, N. and Nielsen, S.L. (1978) Prevalence of primary Raynaud's phenomenon in young females. *Scand. J. Clin. Lab. Invest.*, **38**, 761–70.

Porter, J.M., Bardana, E.J., Baur, G.M., Wesche, D.M., Andrash, R.H. and Rosch, J. (1976) The clinical significance of Raynaud's syndrome. *Surgery*, **80**, 756–64.

Raynaud, M. (1888) Local asphyxia and symmetrical gangrene of the extremities (Translated by Thomas Barlow). In Selected Monographs. The New Sydenham Society, London, p. 99.

Sayre, J.W. (1973) Raynaud's disease presenting in a 5 month old infant. *Pediatrics*, **52**, 412–5.

Spittell, J.A. (1972) in *Peripheral Vascular Diseases* (eds J.F. Fairbanks, J.L. Juergens and J.A. Spittell), W.B. Saunders, Philadelphia, pp. 387–419.

Sumner, D.S. and Strandness, D.E. (1972) An abnormal finger pulse associated with cold sensitivity. *Ann. Surg.*, **175**, 294–8.

Velayos, E.E., Robinson, M., Porcuncula, F.U. and Masi, A. (1971) Clinical correlation analysis of 137 patients with Raynaud's phenomenon. *Am. J. Med. Sci.*, **262**, 347–56.

Zahavi, I., Chagnac, A., Mering, R., Davidovich, S. and Kuritzisy, A. (1984) Prevalence of Raynaud's phenomenon in patients with migraine. *Arch. Intern. Med.*, **144**, 742–4.

3 Haemostasis, haemorheology and Raynaud's phenomenon

JOHN L. FRANCIS and DEBORAH A. FRANCIS

INTRODUCTION

Raynaud's phenomenon (RP) is characterized by reduced blood flow in the peripheral blood vessels which is precipitated or exacerbated by exposure to cold. The small digital arteries and arterioles of patients with severe primary, or scleroderma-associated RP may show intimal proliferation and thrombosis, and in scleroderma, deposits of fibrin may be seen in the lumen of the digital capillaries. As discussed in more detail below, there is evidence of increased blood platelet activation in RP, together with increased levels of some clotting factors and reduced levels of fibrinolytic activity. In addition, patients with RP may show increases in plasma and whole blood viscosity and alterations in red cell deformability have been described. There are close interrelationships between haemostasis and haemorheology, and thus it is possible that these factors, either alone or in combination, may contribute to impaired tissue perfusion and hypercoagulability in RP.

THE HAEMOSTATIC MECHANISM

Haemostasis may be defined as that process which is responsible for the maintenance of the circulating blood in a fluid state and confined to the circulatory system. The haemostatic system is composed of three major components; the blood platelets, the blood coagulation factors and the fibrinolytic pathway. These processes have been extensively reviewed elsewhere and will be discussed only briefly here.

In essence, initial or primary haemostasis is achieved by the adherence of circulating blood platelets to collagen fibres exposed by damage to the endothelial lining of the vessel wall. This process is largely dependent on the presence of von Willebrand factor in the plasma and specific receptor sites on the platelet membrane. Platelet adhesion is rapidly followed by release of some of the platelet contents, including ADP, 5-hydroxytryptamine and products of platelet prostaglandin metabolism. These products stimulate further platelet accumulation at the site of trauma and platelet aggregation. This initial platelet plug limits blood loss from the damaged vessel, but must be reinforced by fibrin, produced by the blood coagulation system, for an impermeable and permanent repair.

The blood coagulation factors are plasma proteins which normally circulate in an inactive form, only becoming active proteolytic enzymes during the process of coagulation. Each activated clotting factor then activates the next protein in the sequence. Exposure to a foreign (i.e. non-endothelial) surface activates the contact factors (factors XII and XI) which trigger the intrinsic coagulation pathway via factors VIII (haemophiliac factor) and IX (Christmas factor). The product of this reaction cleaves factor X, which, in the presence of phospholipid (donated by aggregating platelets), calcium ions and factor V, converts prothrombin into thrombin. The resulting thrombin then converts soluble fibrinogen into an insoluble fibrin clot. Coagulation may also proceed via the extrinsic system in which factor X is activated by factor VII in the presence of tissue factor, a lipoprotein released by tissue damage. Coagulation proceeds very much faster by this pathway, and it is likely that the major function of the extrinsic system is to accelerate, by a series of positive feedback mechanisms, the rate of intrinsic blood coagulation.

After blood coagulation has occurred and tissue repair is underway, the redundant fibrin clot must be removed to restore full patency to the damaged vessel. This is the function of the fibrinolytic system. When fibrin is formed, the elements required for its own ultimate destruction are adsorbed on to the clot from the surrounding plasma. The major component of the fibrinolytic system is the inactive plasma protein, plasminogen. This protein can be converted, by a number of specific activators, into the active enzyme plasmin, the main biological function of which is to break down formed fibrin. Under normal circumstances, this activation is achieved within the fibrin clot by means of tissue plasminogen activator (t-PA), a highly specific activator released into the circulating blood by the endothelial cells of the vessel wall.

It should be noted that a hypercoagulable state (i.e. a condition in which an individual is at greater risk of developing thrombosis) may result from a number of abnormalities of the haemostatic system.

1. Abnormal blood vessel wall structure.
2. Hyperactive blood platelets.
3. Increased levels of blood coagulation factors.
4. Failure of normal inhibitory mechanisms of blood coagulation.
5. Decreased rate of fibrinolysis.
6. Abnormalities of blood flow.

PLATELETS IN RAYNAUD'S PHENOMENON

In view of the association of RP with vascular damage and microthrombosis, much attention has been directed at possible defects of primary haemostasis and their involvement in the vascular lesions of these patients. A variety of abnormalities have been described in patients with peripheral vascular disease, including increased platelet adhesiveness and shortened survival (Murphy and Mustard, 1962), increased platelet aggregation (Ward *et al.*, 1978) and changes in β-thromboglobulin levels (β-TG), platelet production time and plasma heparin neutralizing activity (Cella *et al.*, 1979).

Patients with both primary and secondary forms of RP have also been shown to exhibit enhanced platelet aggregation in response to ADP (Blunt *et al.*, 1980) and adrenaline (Hutton *et al.*, 1984). Platelets from patients with RP generate more thromboxane B_2 than normal after aggregation by ADP, and ADP-induced aggregation is greater at 27°C than at 37°C (Hutton *et al.*, 1984). Patients with RP also have increased numbers of circulating platelet aggregates and raised β-TG concentrations, as well as a greater resistance to the anti-aggregating effects of prostaglandin E_1 and prostacyclin (Hutton *et al.*, 1984). The search for platelet abnormalities induced by cooling *in vivo* has been less rewarding. This may be due to the fact that cooling may result in local platelet activation, but of insufficient magnitude to be detected in the laboratory. Cold can induce platelet aggregation *in vitro* (Kattlove and Alexander, 1971) and hypothermia is associated with an increased incidence of vascular lesions (Mikhailidis *et al.*, 1983). The increased platelet reactivity to various agonists may be a reflection of the increased plasma fibrinogen levels often found in patients with RP (see p. 37). Binding of fibrinogen to platelets is necessary for aggregation to ADP, and increasing fibrinogen concentrations *in vitro* enhances platelet reactivity (Hutton *et al.*, 1984).

It should be noted that cold exposure enhances the vasoconstrictive response to 5-hydroxytryptamine (5-HT) (Vanhoutte and Shepherd, 1970) which is released during the platelet activation process and enhances platelet aggregation to other agents (De Clerck, David and Janssen, 1982). It is therefore of clinical interest that ketanserin, an antagonist of 5-HT, may be beneficial in the treatment of RP (Stranden, Roald and Krohg, 1982).

Most studies of platelet function in RP have not discriminated between primary and secondary forms of this disorder, and there is evidence that those individuals with primary RP have neither increased platelet aggregation *in vivo* nor enhanced aggregation response *in vitro*. Studies in our own laboratories using electrical impedance platelet aggregometry in whole blood have supported this view. There is some evidence however, that 5-HT is a contributory factor in the pathogenesis of RP irrespective of its aetiology (Seibold, 1985). In secondary RP, endothelial cell damage results in continuous *in vivo* platelet activation and 5-HT release. Ketanserin improves blood flow at all temperatures, which suggests the presence of a continuous supply of 5-HT. On the other hand, primary RP is associated with intact endothelium and no increase in platelet activation. In such patients ketanserin does not reduce the frequency of vasospastic attacks, but does effectively relieve cold-induced vasospasm. This suggests that in primary RP, local platelet activation and 5-HT release occur secondarily to vasoconstriction.

Thromboxane A_2, the major cyclooxygenase-derived product of arachidonic acid metabolism in platelets is a powerful vasoconstrictor and potent platelet aggregating agent. Thromboxane synthesis is increased in patients with RP secondary to systemic sclerosis, and may exacerbate cold-induced digital vasospasm (Reilly, Roy and Fitzgerald, 1986).

Overall, there is reasonably strong evidence that platelets play a role in the pathogenesis of secondary RP, although their involvement in the primary form of this disorder remains debatable. Based on this evidence attempts have been made to treat the symptoms of RP with antiplatelet drugs. The results of this approach have, however, been conflicting. The calcium channel blocker nifedipine, inhibits platelet aggregation and has been widely used in the treatment of RP. This drug appears to inhibit *in vivo* platelet activation as evidenced by reduction in plasma β-TG levels (Malamet *et al.*, 1985). However, as nifedipine treatment also reduces the number of vasospastic attacks, it is not clear whether its effect is due to a direct antiplatelet effect, or a secondary effect due to the reduced frequency of vasospasm. The finding that dazoxiben, a thromboxane synthetase inhibitor, is an ineffective treatment (Malamet *et al.*, 1985), suggests that digital vasospasm in RP is not mediated by thromboxane, although an earlier trial (Belch *et al.*, 1983) found dazoxiben to be of some benefit. Although nifedipine does exert an antiplatelet effect, its major effect is presumed to be on the smooth muscle of the digital vessel, and thus it is difficult, if not impossible, to separate the vascular and antiplatelet effects. Similar difficulties are encountered when attempting to interpret the effects of prostacyclin infusion in patients with RP (Belch *et al.*, 1981; Dowd *et al.*, 1982). Ticlopidine, a specific antiplatelet agent which has no vasoactive properties, appears to have no effect on the frequency or severity of Raynaud's attacks, and is therefore evidence against a primary involvement of platelets in the mechanism of RP (Destors *et al.*, 1986).

COAGULATION FACTORS IN RAYNAUD'S PHENOMENON

Patients with both primary and secondary forms of RP have significantly elevated plasma fibrinogen levels (Jarret, Morland and Browse, 1978; Tietjen *et al.*, 1975; Blunt *et al.*, 1980). As detailed above, this may have the effect of enhancing platelet aggregation responses and also results in an increase in the plasma viscosity and rate of red cell aggregation. Any of these effects might be expected to contribute to a hypercoagulable state.

Levels of factor VIII-related antigen (FVIII : RAG) have been shown to be raised in female patients with RP of all aetiologies, although plasma levels of factor VIII clotting activity (FVIII : C) were normal (Blunt *et al.*, 1980). More marked elevations of FVIII : RAG were later reported in both primary RP and scleroderma patients (Kahaleh, Osborn and LeRoy, 1981). Interestingly, similar increases have been observed in patients with diabetes complicated with severe retinopathy, severe atherosclerosis and myocardial infarction; disorders typified by structural vascular disorders. Exposure of patients with scleroderma to cold results in an increase in FVIII : RAG and von Willebrand factor (vWF) activity, and cold injury to endothelial cells *in vitro* stimulates vWF secretion. It remains unclear whether the increased levels favour the development of the vascular lesions, or merely reflect the extent of endothelial injury. Nevertheless, as vWF is involved in the adhesion of blood platelets to the subendothelium, it may play an important role in the development of vascular abnormalities, particularly in patients with scleroderma.

FIBRINOLYSIS IN PATIENTS WITH RAYNAUD'S PHENOMENON

Many patients with primary or scleroderma-related RP have decreased blood fibrinolytic activity as measured by the euglobulin clot lysis time, dilute whole blood clot lysis time or fibrin plate assay (Jarrett, Morland and Browse, 1978). In view of the association of digital fibrin deposition and thrombosis observed in these patients, the possibility of treating the symptoms of RP by pharmacological enhancement of fibrinolysis is clearly attractive. Increased fibrinolysis might be expected to improve hand blood flow either by reducing the plasma fibrinogen levels (and hence blood viscosity) or by degrading intravascular fibrin deposits (and reducing microthrombi formation).

In one double-blind crossover trial, stanozolol administration resulted in a highly significant increase in hand blood flow which persisted after cessation of treatment, and after the plasma fibrinogen levels and fibrinolytic activity had returned to pretreatment levels (Jarrett, Morland and Browse, 1978). Although the mechanism of this effect was not completely elucidated, these investigators concluded that stanozolol should be considered for the treatment of advanced RP when all other methods have failed. Further studies by this group (Ayres, Jarrett and Browse, 1981) showed that although plasma fibrinogen levels were reduced by stanozolol, whole blood viscosity was not.

Thus, the improvement in hand blood flow does not appear to be the result of decreased blood viscosity. The infusion of prostacyclin, as well as having potent vasodilatory and anti-platelet properties, also enhances fibrinolysis (Szczeklik *et al.*, 1983); an effect which is only of clinical benefit when administered in short, 3 h infusions.

HAEMORHEOLOGICAL ABNORMALITIES IN RAYNAUD'S PHENOMENON

There are three major factors which contribute to the viscosity of whole blood: (1) haematocrit; (2) plasma viscosity (plasma protein concentration) and (3) red cell deformability.

Increases in whole blood viscosity in RP have been described by several workers (Pringle, Walder and Weaver, 1965; Walder, 1973; Tietjen *et al.*, 1975; Goyle and Dormandy, 1976; Blunt *et al.*, 1980). The increase in viscosity may be particularly striking when measured under conditions which combine low temperature (27°C) and low shear (Goyle and Dormandy, 1976). Cold provocation of RP by immersion of one hand in cold (4°C) water has been reported to cause a transient increase in blood viscosity, but this finding is not reproducible. Indeed, increase in whole blood viscosity at low temperatures is not specific for RP, and it appears doubtful that patients with primary RP have any evidence of hyperviscosity. The exact cause of the hyperviscosity syndrome of secondary RP has been intensively investigated.

Haematocrit

There is general agreement that patients with RP, irrespective of aetiology, do not exhibit changes in haemoglobin concentration or haematocrit which could account for the increase in whole blood viscosity (Gorjao-Clara, Nunes and Marins-Silva, 1986).

Plasma viscosity

Plasma viscosity is increased in patients with secondary RP (Gorjao-Clara, Nunes and Marins-Silva, 1986). The increase is more pronounced at lower temperatures, and although not confined to RP, this phenomenon might contribute to impaired microvascular perfusion during cooling. Elevations of plasma fibrinogen in RP are well recognized (see p. 33) and usually correlate with the increase in plasma viscosity (Gorjoa-Clara, Nunes and Marins-Silva, 1986). Many patients with RP have a decreased albumen : globulin ratio, (increased serum globulins) and decreased albumen : fibrinogen ratio; factors which predispose to red cell aggregation (Dintenfass, 1977). As might be expected, such patients also have an increased erythrocyte sedimentation rate. Further evidence for a role for elevated plasma viscosity in the pathogenesis of RP has come from successful attempts to relieve the clinical symptoms with repeated plasma exchange (O'Reilly *et al.*, 1979; Weber, Schmid-Schonbein and Lemmens, 1985).

Red cell deformability

As mentioned above, increased whole blood viscosity in RP may be due to elevated plasma viscosity and/or to a reduction in red cell deformability. Although a number of investigators have determined red cell deformability in patients with RP, the results of many early studies must be interpreted with caution. For example, it is difficult to compare results from different studies, as many different methods for the assessment of red cell deformability have been used. In addition, one of the most popular methods for the determination of red cell deformability relies on measuring the rate at which whole blood or red cell suspensions pass through filters of known pore size. These filtration methods are profoundly influenced by the presence of white blood cells, and studies performed before this realization should therefore be discounted.

In a recent report (Bareford *et al.*, 1986), patients with RP were shown to have significant reductions in red cell deformability. This defect is more marked when deformability is assessed with filters having pores of 3 μm diameter, rather than the more commonly used 5 μm filters. In common with viscosity measurements, the abnormality in red cell filterability is more pronounced at lower temperatures, although cold provocation does not further reduce red cell deformability. However, most patients in this study had secondary RP, and studies in this laboratory (Challenor *et al.*, 1987) and those of others (Rustin *et al.*, 1985;

Gorjao-Clara, Nunes and Marins-Silva, 1986) have failed to demonstrate impaired red cell deformability in primary RP.

Red cells from patients with RP associated with systemic sclerosis have been shown to have decreased electrophoretic mobility (Rustin *et al.*, 1985). The exact significance of this finding is unclear, but may reflect alterations in the density of red cell membrane sialic acid residues, or possibly differences in membrane-bound fibrinogen. Patients with primary RP on the other hand, have no such abnormality (Rustin *et al.*, 1985; Smith *et al.*, 1987).

CONCLUSIONS

Interpretation of published data on haemostatic and haemo-rheological changes in patients with RP is difficult. Most studies have not distinguished between primary and secondary forms of the disorder, but it appears that defects of haemostasis and blood flow are largely confined to the secondary group. Further-more, it is difficult to determine whether the blood coagulation and/or fibrinolytic changes give rise to the vascular defects, or are themselves a result of such abnormalities. It is however clear, that from a clinical standpoint, tests of haemostasis and haemorheology are not helpful in the diagnosis of Raynaud's phenomenon, although for reasons stated above, any abnormal-ities are more likely to reflect a secondary cause.

REFERENCES

Ayres, M.L., Jarrett, P.E.M. and Browse, N.L. (1981) Blood viscosity, Raynaud's phenomenon and the effect of fibrinolytic enhancement. *Br. J. Surg.*, **68**, 51–4.
Bareford, D., Coppack, J.S., Stone, P.C.W., Bacon, P.A. and Stuart, J. (1986) Abnormal blood rheology in Raynaud's phenomenon. *Clin. Hemorheol.*, **6**, 53–60.
Belch, J.J.F., Newman, P., Drury, J.K., Capell, H., Lieberman, P., James, W.B., Forbes, C.D. and Prentice, C.R.M. (1981) Successful treatment of Raynaud's syndrome with prostacyclin. *Thrombos. Haemost.*, **45**, 255–6.
Belch, J.J.F., Cormie, J., Newman, P., McLaren, M., Barbenel, J., Capell, H., Lieberman, P., Forbes, C.D. and Prentice, C.R.M. (1983) Dazoxiben, a thromboxane synthetase inhibitor in the treat-ment of Raynaud's syndrome: a double-blind trial. *Br. J. Clin. Pharmacol.*, **15**, 1135–65.

Blunt, R.J., George, A.J., Hurlow, R.A., Strachan, J.L. and Stuart, J. (1980) Hyperviscosity and thrombotic changes in idiopathic and secondary Raynaud's syndrome. *Br. J. Haematol.*, **45**, 651–8.

Cella, G., Zahavi, J., de Haas, H.A. and Kakkar, V.V. (1979) Thrombo-globulin, platelet production time and platelet function in vascular disease. *Br. J. Haematol.*, **43**, 127–36.

Challenor, V.F., Waller, D.G., Francis, D.A., Francis, J.L., Mani, R. and Roath, S. (1987) Nisoldipine in primary Raynaud's phenom-enon. *Eur. J. Clin. Pharmacol.*, (in press).

De Clerk, F.F., David, J.L. and Janssen, P.A.J. (1982) Serotonergic amplification mechanisms in blood platelets. In *5-Hydroxytryptamine in Peripheral Reactions*, (eds F. De Clerk and P.M. Van Houtte), Raven Press, New York, pp. 83–94.

Destors, J.M., Gauthior, E., Lelong, S. and Boissel, J.P. (1986) Failure of a pure antiplatelet drug to decrease the number of attacks more than placebo in patients with Raynaud's phenomenon. *Angiology*, **37**, 565–9.

Dintenfass, L. (1977) Hemorheological factors in Raynaud's phenom-enon. *Angiology*, **28**, 472–81.

Dowd, P.M., Martin, M.F.R., Cooke, E.D., Bow-Cock, S.A., Jones, R., Dieppe, P.A. and Kirby, J.D.T. (1982) Treatment of Raynaud's phenomenon by intravenous infusion of prostacyclin (PGI_2). *Br. J. Dermatol.*, **106**, 81–9.

Gorjao-Clara, J., Nunes, J. and Marins-Silva, J. (1986) Hemorheological studies in Raynaud's syndrome. *Clin. Hemorheol.*, **6**, 245–50.

Goyle, K.B. and Dormandy, J.A. (1976) Abnormal blood viscosity in Raynaud's phenomenon. *Lancet*, **i**, 1317–18.

Hutton, R.A., Mikhailidis, D.P., Bernstein, R.M., Jeremy, J.Y., Hughes, G.R.V. and Dandona, P. (1984) Assessment of platelet function in patients with Raynaud's syndrome. *J. Clin. Pathol.*, **37**, 182–7.

Jarrett, P.E.M., Morland, M. and Browse, N.L. (1978) Treatment of Raynaud's phenomenon by fibrinolytic enhancement. *Br. Med. J.*, **2**, 523–5.

Kahaleh, M.B., Osborn, I. and LeRoy, E.C. (1981) Increased factor VIII/ von Willebrand factor antigen and von Willebrand factor activity in scleroderma and in Raynaud's phenomenon. *Ann. Int. Med.*, **94**, 482–4.

Kattlove, H.E. and Alexander, B. (1971) The effect of cold on platelets. I Cold-induced platelet aggregation. *Blood*, **38**, 39–48.

Malamet, R., Wise, R.A., Ettinger, W.H. and Wigley, F.M. (1985) Nifedipine in the treatment of Raynaud's phenomenon. *Am. J. Med.*, **78**, 602–8.

Mikhailidis, D.P., Hutton, R.A., Jeremey, J.Y. and Dandona, P. (1983) Hypothermia and pancreatitis. *J. Clin. Pathol.*, **36**, 483–4.

Murphy, E.A. and Mustard, J.F. (1962) Coagulation tests and platelet economy in atherosclerosis and control subjects. *Circulation*, **25**, 114–25.

O'Reilly, M.J.G., Talpos, G., Roberts, V.C., White, J.M. and Cotten, L.T. (1979) Controlled trial of plasma exchange in the treatment of Raynaud's syndrome. *Br. Med. J.*, **1**, 1113–15.

Pringle, R., Walder, D.N. and Weaver, J.P.A. (1965) Blood viscosity and Raynaud's disease. *Lancet*, **i**, 1086–9.

Reilly, I.A.G., Roy, L. and Fitzgerald, G.A. (1986) Biosynthesis of thromboxane in patients with systemic sclerosis and Raynaud's phenomenon. *Br. Med. J.*, **292**, 1037–9.

Rustin, M.H.A., Kovacs, I.B., Sowemimo-Coker, S.O., Maddison, P.J. and Kirby, J.D.T. (1985) Differences in red cell behaviour between patients with Raynaud's phenomenon and systemic sclerosis and patients with Raynaud's disease. *Br. J. Dermatol.*, **113**, 265–72.

Seibold, J.R. (1985) Serotonin and Raynaud's phenomenon. *J. Cardiovasc. Pharmacol.*, **7** (Suppl.7), S95–S98.

Smith, R.E., Jones, D.P., Bowcock, S.A. and Cooke, E.D. (1987) The electrophoretic mobility of erythrocytes from patients wtih primary Raynaud's phenomenon. *Clin. Hemorheol.*, **7**, 351–5.

Stranden, E., Roald, O.K. and Krohg, K. (1982) Treatment of Raynaud's phenomenon with the $5HT_2$-receptor antagonist ketanserin. *Br. Med. J.*, **285**, 1069–71.

Szczeklik, A., Kopec, M., Sladek, K., Musial, J., Chmieleswka, J., Teisseyre, E., Dudek-Wojciechowska, G. and Palester-Chlebow-czyk, M. (1983) Prostacyclin and the fibrinolytic system in ischaemic vascular disease. *Thromb. Res.*, **29**, 655–60.

Tietjen, G.W., Chien, S., Leroy, E.C., Gavras, I., Gavras, H. and Gump, F.E. (1975) Blood viscosity, plasma proteins and Raynaud's syndrome. *Arch. Surg.*, **110**, 1343–6.

Vanhoutte, P.M. and Shepherd, J.T. (1970) Effect of temperature on reactivity of isolated cutaneous veins of the dog. *Am. J. Physiol.*, **218**, 187–90.

Walder, D.N. (1973) Blood viscosity and Raynaud's disease. *J. R. Coll. Surg.*, 18, 277–80.

Ward, A.S., Porter, N., Preston, F.E. and Morris-Jones, W. (1978) Platelet aggregation in patients with peripheral vascular disease. *Atherosclerosis*, **29**, 63–8.

Weber, H., Schmid-Schonbein, H. and Lemmens, H.A.J. (1985) Plasma-pheresis as a treatment of Raynaud's attacks: microrheological differential diagnosis and evaluation of efficacy. *Clin. Hemorheol.*, **5**, 85–97.

4 Non-invasive investigations of blood flow in Raynaud's

RAJ MANI

INTRODUCTION

The previous chapters have discussed the prevalence as well as the clinical signs and symptoms which are said to be characteristic of Raynaud's phenomenon (RP). The blood vessels said to be most commonly affected in RP are the digital arterioles (Jurgens, 1983). The effect of the environment on the fingers of patients with RP is said to be one of constriction. If this is the case, digital blood flow in the chronic phase may be expected to be lower than normal. In any acute phase, it may be that not only blood flow but also nutrient transport to the dermal tissues may be affected since patients have digital ulcers on rare occasions.

It has also been stated that when the bluish discolouration of the affected digits is prolonged, there may be 'stasis' in the capillaries and, perhaps the venules in the affected digits (Jurgens, 1983).

'Stasis' is a term used to describe the abnormal concentration of red blood corpuscles. Several early studies of the microcirculation have shown the development of stasis in the tongue and mesentery of the frog and have reported that the obstruction of the venous end of a capillary by closely packed corpuscles is the first stage (Krog, 1929). It also appears that once stasis has occurred, it is generally irreversible, although the resolution of stasis in the capillaries in the rat mesentery has been reported. Ryan (1974) has suggested that the effect of cold on the fluid properties of blood which allow it to flow may also aid in the development of stasis. Thus it would appear that pathological as well as haemorheological events may precipitate the development of RP. Objective diagnostic techniques should therefore, be capable of identifying and discriminating any pathological vascular and/or haemorheological changes that are said to occur in patients with RP. This chapter is devoted to the potential offered by a number of techniques to achieve this objective. It needs to be emphasized at the outset that the author is not aware of any technique being routinely used in vascular laboratories as an aid in the clinical management of RP.

The potentials of non-invasive and therefore, indirect, techniques to measure microcirculatory disturbances are critically appraised in this chapter.

TECHNIQUES

There are at least five techniques which are potentially useful for the clinical investigation of RP. These are microscopy, photoplethysmography, laser Doppler flowmetry, ultrasound Doppler flowmetry and finally radioisotope clearance technique.

Microscopy

A common binocular microscope with a magnification of × 25 to × 40 allows the capillaries in the nailfold of fingers and toes to be visualized. An ordinary tungsten filament bulb can be used as the light source although when a green filter is interposed between the source and the nailbed visualization of blood corpuscles is easier. A drop of any light oil on the nailbed serves to minimize refraction effects and the author has found plain, wet nail varnish to be effective in this respect.

It has been reported by Mariq (1980) that only 9% (1/11) of patients with RP had dilated and tortuous vessels with avascular areas in the nailfold. The study does not suggest that the technique has any diagnostic potential for RP.

There is some similarity between the observations of tortuosity and loss of vessels or 'drop out' in Mariq's study and those in the studies of Leu (1965), Fagrell (1979) and Ryan (1974) who were studying the legs of patients with chronic venous incompetence. These latter workers are, at present, the major protagonists of stasis in the development of venous disease and ulcers.

The advent of low-light-level television cameras has made it possible to visualize and measure capillary flow velocities in nailfolds (Tooke and Milligan, 1983) of patients with haematological disturbances such as some leukaemias. No such studies on RP have been reported to the author's knowledge. The advantage of the microscopy technique is its simplicity. Although television or videomicroscopy is likely to get cheaper, its availability is, at present, limited to one centre in the UK. Further studies are required before the value of this technique is known but at present, it offers attractive potential.

Photoplethysmography

Of the techniques available to study cutaneous blood flow, photoplethysmography is historically the first, having been reported by Hertzman in 1938. The technique is extremely simple and is based on the reflection and absorption of light by tissues. The proportion of incident light not absorbed by tissues is reflected. This reflected fraction is modulated by the blood pulse waveform and simple electronic differentiation enables a trace of the blood volume pulse to be obtained (Challoner, 1973; Roberts, 1981; and Mani and White, 1985). The transducer or probe can be developed easily with light-sensitive detectors and emitters which are readily available in the UK. Most probes including those that are commercially available use a small white light source which costs on average £1000 ($1500). The author has designed a probe using infrared sources and detectors for cutaneous work (Mani and White, 1985). The use of infrared sources has only been possible in recent years and offers the advantage of greater penetration than other wavelengths. Infrared sources which are capable of sensing movement thus make good probes for detecting pulse volume changes. The other advantage offered by infrared sources is that they can be used without interference from ambient lighting. The major limitation of photoplethysmography is that *in vivo* calibration is not possible. Since tissue scatters and absorbs light in a complex manner and since tissue comprises many constituents with differing and largely unknown optical properties, it has not been possible to model the optical behaviour of tissue adequately. Consequently, photoplethysmographs have to be compared with other and older techniques capable of making the same measurement in order to assess relative reproducibility. The photoplethysmograph developed by the author and colleagues has a coefficient of variation of 3.8–4.5% on the forearm and back, respectively, of resting normal subjects which suggests that the system is fairly free of 'noise'. When used to measure the cutaneous vascular responses to intradermal injections of inflammatory mediators, it was found to be sensitive enough to discriminate between individuals receiving histamine and controls, although not specific enough to identify the responses to individual dosages of histamine (Hovell, 1986). The photoplethysmograph is not capable of differentiating the direction of flow and can register increases in blood volume only. The author has successfully used it to detect cutaneous pulsatility around leg ulcers (Mani and White, 1984, 1985). In a clinical trial to assess the response of a group ($n = 40$) with primary Raynaud's to nisoldipine, the author was unable to distinguish different responses to digital artery occlusion between individual patients or groups using this photoplenthysmograph. However, there were no significant changes in other parameters such as red cell deformability or clinical benefit from this therapy either.

In conclusion, photoplethysmography is a simple technique that could be easily available even to the family practitioner but the technique will only grossly detect the presence or absence of cutaneous pulsatility. Sophisticated computer software does allow the analysis of such cutaneous pulsatility but not for the purpose of measuring blood volume since, as stated, photoplethysmography is not direction sensitive.

Laser Doppler flowmetry

Stern (1975) reported that the backscatter from coherent light could be used to study the microcirculation. Nilsson (1984) and Bonner (1981) working independently but at the same time developed the laser Doppler flowmeter. The apparatus developed by Nilsson is manufactured by Perimed. The Bonner development has been commercially exploited by Medpacific Inc. and at the time of writing, is not available in the UK.

Laser Doppler systems use a low-power helium neon tube

which emits red light that is coupled to a small (3mm diameter) probe via fibre-optic connectors. Tenland (1982) has suggested that the Perimed laser detects blood flow at depths up to 1 mm in skin, and that this laser Doppler system is capable of measuring changes in blood-flow reliably. The author's experience confirms this (Hovell, 1987).

The laser Doppler assessment is sensitive to volume flow as well as direction. Nilsson (1984) claims that the system detects 'velocity and number of scattering particles, i.e. red blood cells' in the sample volume which is said to be approximately $1.5 \, mm^3$ (Tenland, 1982). In the author's understanding the laser Doppler detects the redness as well as the pulsatility of the cutaneous vasculature. Watkins and Holloway (1978) experimentally showed a close association ($r^2 = 0.87$) between laser Doppler flowmetry and xenon clearance while studying blood flow in the skin of the foot. There is a small school of critics who maintain that the xenon clearance does not measure blood flow but some parameter related to blood flow which might question the findings of Watkins and Holloway although there is no doubt about the validity of the correlation expressed in their work. Tooke, Oestergen and Fagrell (1983) measured capillary blood flow using capillary microscopy, laser Doppler flowmetry and skin temperature measurements and suggested that these techniques may not be measuring flow in the same vessels.

We have used laser Doppler flowmetry (Periflux PFIC, Perimed, Sweden) to measure resting blood flow in the finger nailbed of patients ($n = 36$) with RP. The patients studied were on a double-blind study of nifedipine. There was no significant association with therapeutic benefits obtained in a small number and nailbed blood flow.

There is little doubt that the laser Doppler detects cutaneous vascular responses reliably and reproducibly (Cole, Mani and Sedgwick, 1985; Mani and Beaseley, 1987). Failure to discriminate between patients with RP from normal controls may be attributed to lack of dissimilarity between groups in the resting condition. For this reason, it may be necessary to carry out provocative challenges involving cooling of the body or a digit. Whichever of the provocative techniques is ultimately most successful, it will require a thermally stable and well-controlled environment in which it can be carried out.

Ultrasound techniques

Doppler ultrasound offers a reliable means of detecting blood flow and has been clinically used for detecting arterial occlusive and stenotic diseases as well as venous thrombosis. The principle was first enunciated by Johann Christian Doppler in 1793. In essence, a moving particle sets up pressure waves which move faster toward the observer when the particle is moving toward him. On the contrary, the pressure waves are slower when the moving particle is receding from the observer. The change in frequency or 'frequency shift' is given by the formula $df = 2fx \cos \theta / v$ where v = velocity of ultrasound in that medium, f = frequency of insonation and θ is the angle of insonation. The factor $\cos\theta$ makes a major contribution to the Doppler shift obtained and can be demonstrated by altering the angle made by the Doppler probe with skin surface. The biggest Doppler

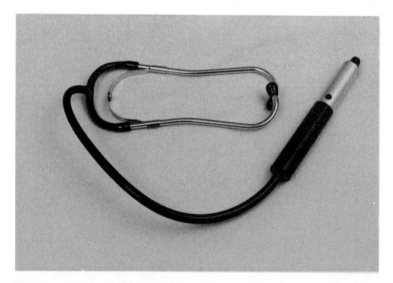

Fig. 4.1 Simple 4MHz Doppler ultrasound stethoscope (Huntleigh Technology 501)

shift is obtained when the ultrasound beam travels at 0° to the direction of flow, in other words towards it along the artery.

The electronic differentiation of forward from reverse flow is more or less routine these days and the technique is used widely as a screening test in the UK to detect arterial and deep venous problems. In practice, a coupling medium such as Acquasonic[R] gel is needed to transmit the ultrasound in to the body. The choice of probe is governed by the vessel to be studied, the higher frequency probe being less capable of penetration is therefore selected for more superficial or subcutaneous vessels. The author has used a simple 4 MHz Doppler ultrasound 'stethoscope' (Huntleigh Technology 501) (Fig. 4.1) to detect digital artery patency in RP. The system is safe, simple and has reliably detected digital artery patency with an accuracy of 100%.

An example of digital artery flow in the forefinger of a patient who complained that her fingers went 'blue with cold' is shown in Fig. 4.2. The figure shows the three components of flow in a normal pulsatile artery when detected by Doppler using elec-

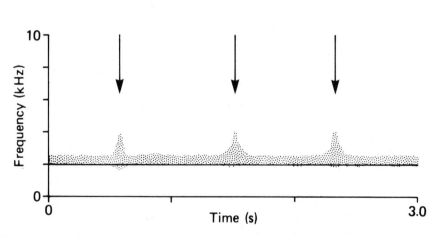

Fig. 4.2   Three components of flow in a normal pulsatile digital artery detected by Doppler using electronic differentiation

tronic differentiation to extract the maximum frequency of Doppler shift. At present, Doppler ultrasound techniques do not offer useful data to the physician treating a patient with RP although, in this author's opinion, with improved technology, real-time ultrasound probes may be available to image digital arteries and veins.

Radioisotope clearance techniques

The first technique was described by Kety (1948), who reported that when an easily diffusible radioisotope tracer in a bolus of saline was injected intravenously, intradermally or intra-arterially the clearance of the tracer from the region was a quantifiable measure of the local blood flow. This clearance could be expressed as a logarithmic decay and since the rate of decay of an isotope is one of its characteristics, the blood flow can be calculated. The time taken by an isotope to decay to 50% of its initial activity is called its biological 'half-life'. The technique hinges on the fundamental assumption that the radioisotope tracer 'labels' blood cells, thus allowing the rate of blood flow to be measured.

For studies of skin blood flow sodium (^{24}Na), xenon (^{133}Xe), technetium (molybdenum pertechnetate) and 4-iodoantipyrine (^{125}I) are all useful as tracers. In order to study blood flow in a digit, the chosen isotope can be injected or allowed to diffuse transcutaneously although only xenon can be used in the latter case. The radioactivity in the blood can be detected by a sodium iodide crystal that is sensitive to radioactivity together with a counter and recorder. When using xenon and technetium, a 'gamma camera' or a counter sensitive to gamma energy can be used to measure the decay of the injected radioactive dose. Sodium is not very suitable for most studies since the clearance of the sodium molecule is dependent on the metabolic activity in the region. Xenon has the advantage of a very short half-life of 30 s which allows repeat measurements to be made. All isotopes cling to fat particles which cause signal-to-noise problems. McCollum and Spence (1985) are of the view that ^{125}I is the least 'noisy' in this context. In the same report Spence has suggested that this property of ^{125}I together with careful methodology may be the primary reasons for their repeatable and reliable results of blood flow in ischaemic skin.

It is also possible to study capillary perfusion by injecting radioactively labelled microspheres (15–50 μm in diameter) intra-arterially thus causing the microspheres to be trapped in capillary beds. The radioactive counts and the subsequent decay can be detected and measured by methods similar to those for the injection technique.

The main limitation of the radioisotope-clearance technique is the need for a nuclear medicine department with its specialized skills.

CHALLENGE TESTS

There are references in the literature to successful methods of measuring changes in digital blood flow in RP which use provocation (Creager *et al.*, 1984). Creager has reported measuring increased finger blood-flow in eight out of ten patients taking nifedipine although the overall change in flow (7.9 ± 3.5 to 7.5 ± 2.1 ml/100ml/min) was not statistically significant. Creager used air plethysmography, a very expensive, sophisticated technique, to achieve their findings.

DISCUSSIONS AND RECOMMENDATIONS

The lack of success of any technique and methodology in measuring changes in digital flow in RP may to a certain extent be a reflection of the difficulties faced in mimicking a genuine Raynaud's attack. Future technological innovations may permit the microcirculation to be studied with high precision and when such advances are available, the kinetics of changes induced by 'challenges' or provocations may need close examination. At present, a portable Doppler probe offers at best a simple objective means which can also be widely available for documenting digital artery patency.

REFERENCES

Bonner, R.F., Roders, G.R. and Schecter, A.W. (1981) Laser Doppler velocimeter and number density of flowing red blood cells in sickle cell anaemia. *Int. J. Microcirc. Clin. Exp.*, **3**, 432.
Challoner, A.V.J. (1973) PhD Thesis, University of London.
Cole, J., Mani, R. and Sedgwick, E.M. (1985) Cutaneous vasomotor reflexes following spinal injury in man. *J. Physiol.*, **3**, 134P, 369.

Creager, M.A., Parsen, K.M. *et al.* (1984) Nifedipine induced fingertip vasodilation in patients with Raynaud's phenomenon *Am. Heart. J.*, **108**(2), 370–3.

Fagrell, B. (1979) Local microcirculation in chronic venous incompetence and leg ulcers. *Vasc. Surg.*, **13**, 217–23.

Hovell, C.J. (1986) PGD_2 is an inflammatory mediator with vascular effects in human skin. BM Thesis, University of Southampton.

Hovell, C.J., Beasley, C.R.W., Mani, R. and Holgate, S.T. (1987) Laser Doppler flowmetry for determining changes in cutaneous blood flow following intradermal injections of histamine. *Clin. Allergy*, **17**(5).

Jurgens, J.L., Spittell, J.A. and Fairbairn, J.F. (1983) *Peripheral Vascular Diseases*. Saunders, New York.

Kety, S.S. (1948) Quantitative measurement of regional circulation by the clearance of radioactive sodium. *Am. J. Med. Sci.*, **215**, 352–3.

Krog, A. (1929) *The Anatomy and Physiology of Capillaries*. Yale University Press, Connecticut, USA.

Leu, H.J. (1965) The prognostic significance of cutaneous and microvascular changes in venous leg ulcers. *Vasc. Dis.*, **2**, 77.

Mani, R. and White, J.E. (1984) A methodology for studying leg ulcers. *Int. J. Microcirc. Clin. Exp.*, **2**, 277–83.

Mani, R. and White, J.E. (1985) The use of photoreflectance probes and transcutaneous oxygen electrodes for investigations of leg ulcers. *Bioeng. Skin*, **1**, 207–13.

Mani, R. and Beasley, C.R.W. (1987) Can cutaneous vascular responses be measured? *Anglo Dutch Thermographic Soc.*, (in press).

Mariq, H.R., Lewry, E.C., D'Angelo, W.A., Medsger, T.A., Rodnam, G.D., Sharp, G.C. and Wolfe, J.F. (1980) Diagnostic potential of *in vivo* capillary microscopy in scleroderma and related disorders. *Arthritis Rheumatol.*, **23**, 183–9.

McCollum, P.T., Spence, V.A. and Walker, W.F. (1985) Circumferential skin blood flow measurements in the ischaemic limb. *Br. J. Surg.*, **72**, 310–12.

Nilsson, G.E. (1984) Signal processor for laser Doppler tissue flowmeters. *IEEE Trans BME*, 343–7.

Roberts, V.C. (1982) Photoplethysmography – fundamental aspects of the optical properties of blood in motion. *Trans. Inst. Meas. Control*, **4**, 317–28.

Ryan, T.J. (1974) *Microvascular Injury*. Academic Press, London.

Stern, M.D. (1975) *In vivo* evaluation of microcirculation by coherent light scattering. *Nature*, **254**, 56–8.

Tenland, T. (1982) *On laser Doppler flowmetry*. Linkoping studies in Science and Technology Dissertations no 83, University of Linkoping, Sweden.

Tooke, J. and Milligan, D. (1983) Capillary flow velocity in leukaemia. *Br. Med. J.*, **286**, 518–9.

Tooke, J., Oestergen, T. and Fagrell, B. (1983) Synchronous assessment of skin microcirculation by laser Doppler flowmetry and dynamic capillaroscopy. *Int. J. Microcirc. Clin. Exp.*, **2**, 277–83.

Watkins, D.W. and Holloway, G.A. (1978) An instrument to measure cutaneous blood flow using the Doppler shift of laser light. *IEEE Trans. BME*, **25**, 28–33.

5 *Sensory aspects of Raynaud's phenomenon*

ROBERT HAYWARD and MICHAEL GRIFFIN

SENSORY FUNCTIONS OF THE SKIN

The glabrous skin of the human hand, particularly that at the fingertips, is richly innervated with sensory nerve endings. These nerve endings provide us with a wide variety of information about our world; its temperature, its texture, its softness or hardness, its shape, form and size. In persons suffering from Raynaud's phenomenon, the fingertip skin containing these sensory receptors will experience attacks of vasospasm. This chapter examines whether there are changes in sensory functions among those with Raynaud's phenomenon. Such changes might occur either as a consequence of vasospasm or by a disorder of the neurological control of circulation.

Sensory receptors in the skin respond to a variety of stimuli. There may be over 15 morphologically and functionally different end-organs in the skin (Iggo, 1982). There are three main classes of these end-organs:

1. Nociceptors, or pain receptors, with unencapsulated 'free' nerve endings, respond to intense mechanical stimulation or to extreme temperatures. These receptors do not show any activity during normal conditions.
2. Thermoceptors, or temperature receptors, are of two types, 'warm' receptors and 'cold' receptors. These respond to skin temperatures deviating from body temperature.
3. The largest group of end-organs in the skin are mechano-receptors. These respond to pressure and indentation of the skin and are responsible for the 'feel' of the world. There are two main types of mechanoreceptors, slowly adapting and rapidly adapting. Slowly adapting receptors such as Merkel cells and Ruffini endings are sensitive to constantly maintained pressure

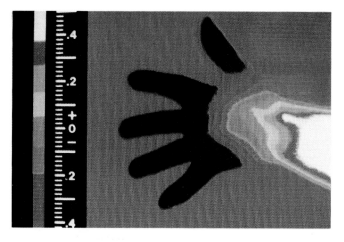

Plate 1 Thermogram showing typically cold fingers in a patient with Raynaud's phenomenon showing all of the digits symmetrically involved

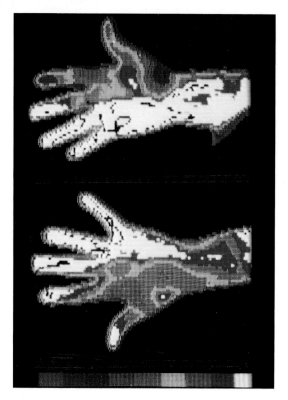

Plate 2 Thermogram of a Raynaud's patient showing asymmetrical coldness in approximately half of the hand

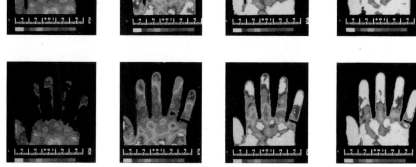

Plate 3 A sequence of thermograms taken at 20s intervals after cold stress in the hand of a healthy subject. The thermal recovery for the palmar surface occurs in a characteristic sequence, which includes the opening of the digital vessels followed by the arteriovenous anastomosis

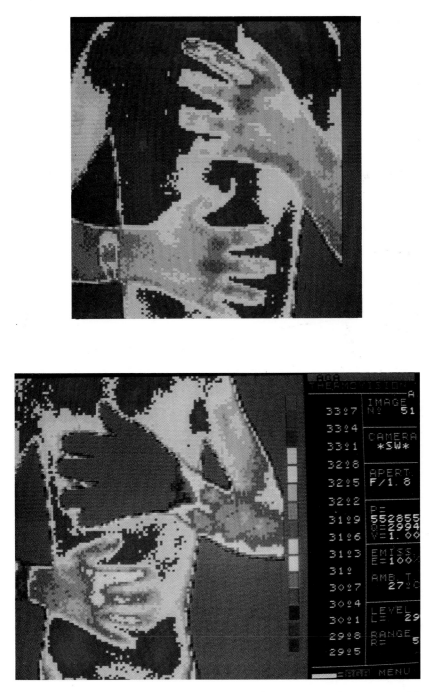

Plate 4 UPPER Precold stress thermogram of the hands of a 14-year-old boy with a cold left index finger (see text). LOWER Cooling of the index finger of the right hand in response to cold stress of the left hand

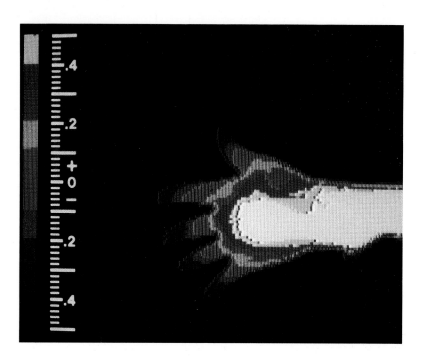

Plate 5 ABOVE Temperature pattern over a Raynaud's patient with coldness in all the digits. UPPER RIGHT Thermogram of the same hand covered by an electrically heated glove just prior to electric heating; LOWER RIGHT Temperature pattern over the electrically heated glove after some ten minutes of use

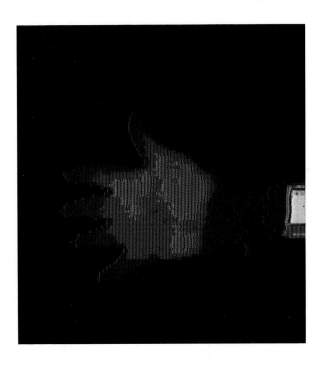

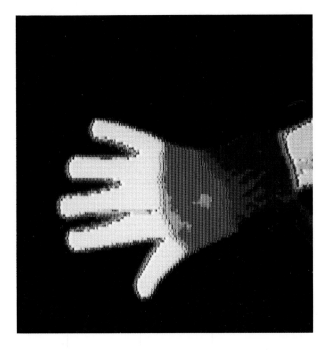

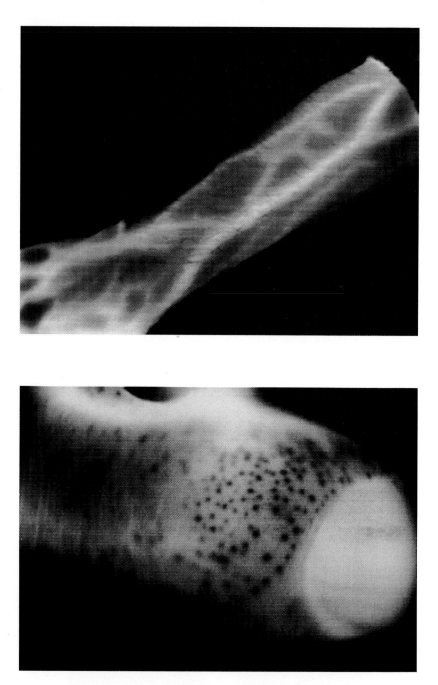

Plate 6   High resolution thermograms produced by the Rank Prize Fund thermal scanner. UPPER Vascular patterns over the forearm visualized in considerable detail. LOWER Individual sweat pores on the fingers showing up as dark, well-defined spots

on the skin, and to gradual changes of indentation or pressure. Rapidly adapting mechanoreceptors do not respond to constant force, only to changes in force; they are thus velocity or acceleration sensitive whereas slowly adapting receptors are displacement sensitive. Rapidly adapting receptors are particularly suited to detect mechanical vibration.

In glabrous skin, rapidly adapting receptors, called Meissner corpuscles, lie in the dermal papillae within the raised epidermal ridges (Quilliam, 1978). These respond to mechanical vibrations of frequencies in the approximate range 5–60 Hz with maximal response around 20–40 Hz. Far deeper in the skin (around 3 mm below the skin surface) lie Pacinian corpuscles. These are highly specialized receptors whose laminated encapsulation ensures that they will not fire in response to any stimuli other than high frequency indentation. They respond to a wide

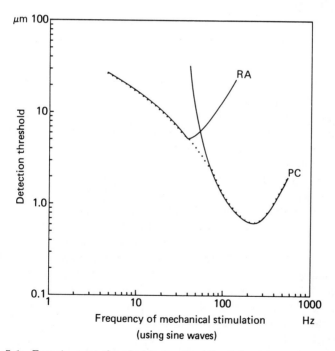

Fig. 5.1 Entrainment thresholds for Rapidly Adapting and Pacinian afferent fibres from the glabrous skin of the monkey. (Adapted from Iggo, 1982.) (PC = Pacinian, RA = rapidly adapting)

range of frequencies (50–1000 Hz) but are only highly sensitive to a narrow range of frequencies, approximately 100–300 Hz. Figure 5.1 shows an idealized representation of the detection thresholds of rapidly adapting receptors, and the corresponding psychophysical perception thresholds.

The function of these receptors specialized for the perception of vibration stimuli can be understood if the sense of touch is seen as active rather than passive. The use of the hand to explore the edges and textures of the world provides vibratory stimuli to the fingers (Katz, 1925; Gordon, 1978). It is a complex interaction of signals from different types of mechanoreceptive units and from proprioceptive receptors in the hands that gives rise to the sensations of touch that we experience. Slowly adapting mechanoreceptors tell us much of the basic form of the world, but it is thought that the rapidly adapting mechano-receptors yield the sensation of fine touch associated with details and textures.

VIBROTACTILE PERCEPTION: METHODS AND PROBLEMS

Various tests of tactile sensation have been used in clinical and experimental work to evaluate sensory loss in a variety of disorders. These range from simple 'uncontrolled' clinical tests, to see if the patient can feel a pin-prick, brushing with cotton wool or the vibrations from a tuning fork, to more quantifiable methods such as depth sense, two-point discrimination and temperature sense (Kenshalo, 1970).

The perception of vibration from a tuning fork has been employed in neurology for at least a century (Rumpf, 1889). The development of methods of producing vibration electrically has allowed more precise and easy control of the stimulus and psychophysical studies have been carried out for many years. Knudsen (1928) and Geldard (1940) provide reviews of much of the early work. The ease of the method has led to its use in clinical investigations of patients with various disorders and devices for measuring vibrotactile perception thresholds have been developed (Sallé and Verbank, 1984; Goldberg and Lind-blom, 1979).

In developing apparatus for use in the evaluation of patients with vibration-induced white finger and primary Raynaud's disease, the present authors have attempted to reduce the variability in measurements. Such variability may arise from inadequate control of the test method, variability within subjects at different test times, and variability between subjects other than that attributable to the condition of interest.

Psychophysical studies have shown that the configuration of the apparatus used will affect threshold measures. The area of contact with vibration, the force of the contact and the presence of a fixed surround will all have an influence (Verrillo, 1966). It is necessary to standardize these factors. A simple way to ensure constant force on the finger is to mount the vibrator assembly on a counter-balanced beam; the use of a fixed surround helps to control the posture of the finger (Fig. 5.2). To control the test method further, the force of the finger downwards upon the fixed surround can be controlled by showing the subject a meter indicating the force as measured by strain gauges on the surrounding plate. The control of the level of the stimulus is automated by the use of a microcomputer. In the apparatus developed by the authors, an up–down method of limits was used to obtain threshold measures, with the stimulus intensity

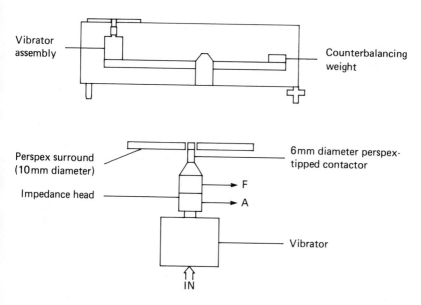

Fig. 5.2 Apparatus to measure vibrotactile thresholds

being increased until the patient signalled that they could feel the vibration (by means of a hand-held response button) and then being decreased until it could no longer be felt.

The existence of two populations of rapidly adapting receptors suggested that it would be appropriate to determine thresholds at two frequencies so that the functions of each receptor type could be assessed. Using the apparatus with normal subjects the variation of threshold with frequency differed slightly from person to person (Fig. 5.3 and Hayward, 1986). However, in all cases there appeared to be a clear discontinuity at around 50 Hz (see Fig. 5.1). The threshold measures at 31.5 Hz and 125 Hz appear differentially to test the two receptor populations.

In carrying out the test it is first necessary to provide the patient with an initial 'practice' measurement. Following this, repeatable and reproducible results may be expected (Hayward, 1986). As skin temperatures will influence thresholds (Green, 1977; Weitz, 1941) it is important to measure skin temperature prior to measuring vibrotactile perception. This is particularly necessary in patients with circulatory disorders, where it is wished to ascribe changes in threshold to underlying physiological causes, rather than to the fact that such patients tend to have cold fingers. With the apparatus it appears that thresholds free from such artefacts can be obtained if the finger temperature is greater than 20°C at the time of the test (Hayward and Griffin, 1986).

Substantial vibration exposures will cause a temporary elevation of thresholds. In consequence, where Raynaud's phenomenon has an occupational cause (vibration-induced white finger) vibrotactile sensation must not be measured until this effect has disappeared following vibration work (Hayward and Griffin, 1986; Hayward, 1986).

Various medical conditions other than Raynaud's phenomenon may influence thresholds. These include many neurological conditions, diabetes, scleroderma and injuries to the hands, arms, shoulders and neck. Both patients and controls should be screened to identify individuals whose thresholds may be affected by such conditions.

In a control population screened for medical conditions, there is an elevation of threshold with age (Fig. 5.4). This relationship can be used to provide an expected threshold for a patient of any age. In comparing patients with controls an age-weighted thres-

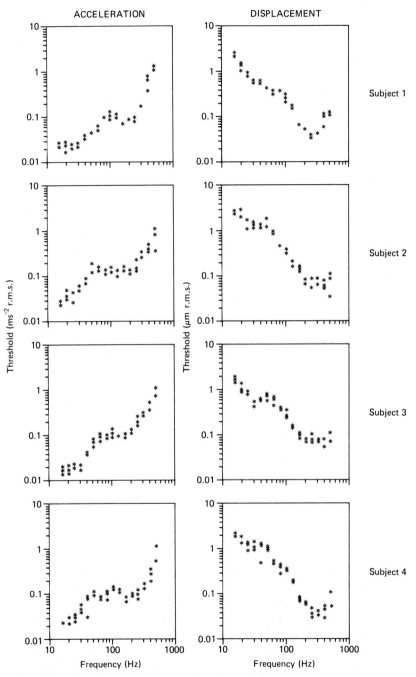

Fig. 5.3 Frequency functions of vibrotactile thresholds for four subjects

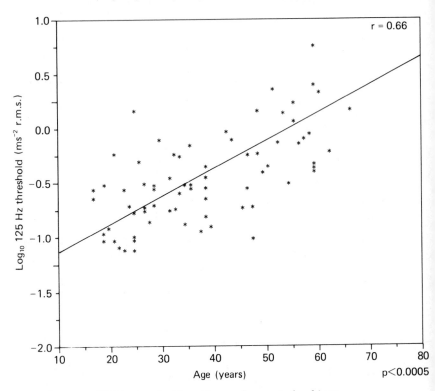

Fig. 5.4   125 Hz thresholds with age for control subjects

hold can be employed. There do not appear to be significant differences in threshold between male and female subjects.

VIBROTACTILE THRESHOLDS IN PERSONS OCCUPATIONALLY EXPOSED TO VIBRATION

Vibration-induced white finger (VWF) is a form of secondary Raynaud's phenomenon caused by occupational exposure to hand-transmitted vibration. It may occur in workers using a variety of tools, primarily in persons using chain-saws, percussive tools such as chipping-hammers and rock drills or metalworking tools such as hand-held and pedestal grinders or polishers. Depending on tool type, the prevalence of the disorder among workers can vary from a few per cent to 100%; the period of time between commencing vibration-exposure and developing symptoms may be as low as 6 months or may be greater than 20 years.

Vibration-induced white finger typically manifests itself as attacks of blanching of the fingers in response to cold. The disorder is progressive, with blanching originally affecting only the tips of one or two fingers and occurring only occasionally. If vibration exposure is continued, the extent of the blanching will increase, and attacks become more frequent. In severe cases cyanosis and necrosis may eventually develop.

Vibration-induced white finger is not the only result of occupational exposure to hand–arm vibration. Bone and joint disorders (bone cysts, arthritic conditions etc.) are reported, mainly from the use of percussive tools and muscular and neurological problems have been detected in persons using a wide range of tool types (Griffin, 1982).

The diagnosis of VWF, like the diagnosis of primary Raynaud's disease, is made problematic by the episodic nature of the disorder, and the difficulty of provoking attacks during an examination. The medical–legal aspects of the disorder (VWF became a prescribed industrial disease in Britain in 1985), make it especially desirable to have an objective indicator of the severity of the disease. Tests of circulatory function (e.g. Olsen and Nielsen (1979) – blood flow during cooling; Harada and Matsumoto (1984) – finger temperature before and after cooling) have been evaluated, although it is unclear whether any are sufficiently accurate for diagnostic purposes at an individual level.

The use of vibrotactile thresholds as a diagnostic test has been evaluated (e.g. Pelmear *et al.*, 1975; Aatola *et al.*, 1982). The results of these investigations have tended to show some elevation of threshold above normal in persons with VWF, but an accurate assessment of the diagnostic potential of the test cannot be made on the basis of these results. Most studies have investigated small groups of individuals, and have often compared the thresholds of patients with VWF against those of non-exposed workers, rather than assessed the ability of the test to discriminate between vibration-exposed workers with and without VWF.

One reason for thinking that vibrotactile thresholds may prove a diagnostic test for VWF is that neurological symptoms (tingling and numbness of the fingers) have often been thought to occur in patients prior to the development of blanching, and this is assumed by the classification of severity prepared by Taylor and Pelmear (1975). However, in the vibration-exposed workers studied by these authors this relationship is not clearly seen – around 20% of patients with VWF reported neurological symptoms appearing after the first onset of blanching, or not at all.

It is now clear that vibration exposure leads to elevated vibrotactile perception thresholds, and that this elevation occurs for perception mediated by both types of vibrotactile end-organs. In populations of 215 metal workers and 146 chain-saw operators most vibration-exposed workers had elevated thresholds (Hayward and Griffin, in preparation). However, the difference between vibration-exposed workers with and without VWF was very small (although still statistically significant) as shown in Fig. 5.5 and 5.6 for 125 Hz thresholds. The small difference between those with and without VWF may arise because those with VWF will tend to have experienced more vibration exposure,

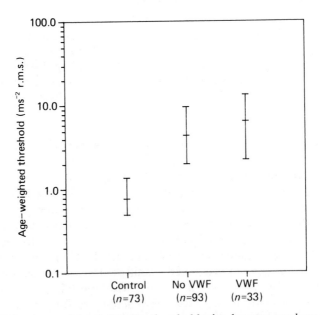

Fig. 5.5 Age-weighted 125 Hz thresholds for forestry workers with and without blanching compared to a control group not exposed to vibration

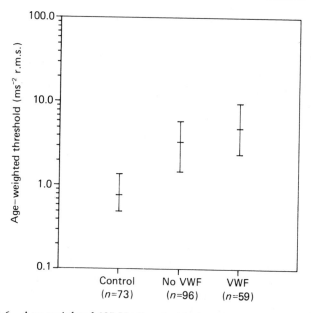

Fig. 5.6 Age-weighted 125 Hz thresholds for metal-workers with and without blanching compared to a control group not exposed to vibration

and this exposure will influence their thresholds. The difficulty of accurately quantifying vibration exposure over many years precludes a true evaluation of this expectation. Similarly the relationships between VWF and exposure or vibrotactile thresholds and exposure are difficult to establish. It is possible that VWF causes some elevation of thresholds, but that this is small compared to the direct effect of the vibration exposure.

It is concluded that vibration exposure causes elevated vibrotactile thresholds as well as VWF. The evidence of the present authors would suggest that these two effects are primarily unrelated and that while increased vibration exposure makes it more likely that both effects occur, individual predisposition to damage may result in some persons developing VWF without significant impairment of sensory function, while others may show marked threshold elevation without symptoms of circulatory disorder.

VIBROTACTILE THRESHOLDS IN PATIENTS WITH PRIMARY RAYNAUD'S DISEASE

The results of the investigations of vibration-exposed workers suggested that there was little relation between vibrotactile sensitivity and circulatory disorder. However, in a control group not exposed to vibration, some subjects were found who showed symptoms of other forms of Raynaud's phenomenon. As these subjects showed thresholds somewhat elevated above the normal (Table 5.1), it was of interest to investigate whether vibrotactile thresholds had any application to the evaluation of primary Raynaud's disease.

Patients with primary Raynaud's disease do not show the large sensory loss seen in many vibration-exposed workers. However, there is some evidence of elevated thresholds in the 36 patients so far evaluated (Figures 5.7 and 5.8). The degree of elevation is not sufficient to diagnose the existence of the condition – only 12 out of 36 patients had 125 Hz thresholds above the 90% threshold of the normal population and only 7 out of 36 met this criterion for 31.5 Hz vibration.

There are no clear features distinguishing those patients with elevated thresholds from those with thresholds in the normal range, the distribution of the thresholds among patients similarly shows no evidence of two distinct groups. However, it appears that elevated thresholds may tend to be associated with more attacks (Fig. 5.9). In patients with infrequent attacks of blanching the thresholds are more likely to remain in the normal range. This might suggest a causal link between blanching and

Table 5.1 Thresholds of control subjects reporting and not reporting finger blanching

	Subjects without blanching (n = 137)	Subjects with blanching (n = 26)
Median 31.5 Hz threshold (ms^{-2} r.m.s.)	0.056	0.067
Median 125 Hz threshold (ms^{-2} r.m.s.)	0.349	0.699

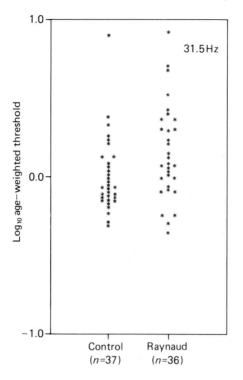

Fig. 5.7 Age-weighted 31.5 Hz thresholds for Raynaud's patients compared to control subjects

elevated thresholds. Repeated ischaemia of the digits may lead to damage of the peripheral nerve endings, and thus to elevated thresholds. However, the finding that thresholds were elevated on all digits of the patients, not just on those affected by blanching, suggests that this may not be a sufficient explanation. It is possible that a common factor underlies both sensory and circulatory problems. This affects peripheral neurological functioning, thus interfering with both sensory function and the neural control of vascular tone. It is not possible to suggest whether the underlying mechanisms of blanching and sensory loss in VWF and primary Raynaud's disease are the same without further evidence – this requires research into both neurological and circulatory functioning in both groups of patients.

Even if vibrotactile thresholds do not provide a diagnostic test

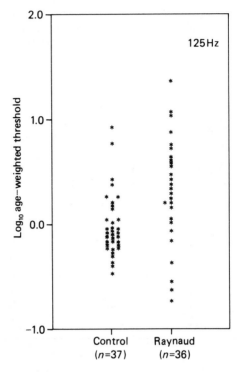

Fig. 5.8 Age-weighted 125 Hz thresholds for Raynaud's patients comared to control subjects

for the existence of primary Raynaud's disease, they may prove a useful indicator of the effectiveness of drug treatments. In a clinical trial of the calcium antagonist nifedipine (Challoner *et al.*, in preparation), although there was no observed effect of the drug on vibration thresholds, the pre-treatment vibrotactile thresholds provided a good indicator of response to the drug (Fig. 5.10). Patients with low thresholds responded well to the treatment whereas patients with elevated thresholds did not receive great benefit. This could be because thresholds are a good indicator of severity (severity being more than just the frequency of attacks as reported by the patient: duration and extent will also be important). Alternatively, this finding may be related to the way in which both the drug and the cause of Raynaud's phenomenon affect the control of circulation.

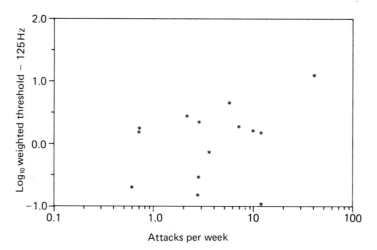

Fig. 5.9 125 Hz thresholds and severity (number of attacks per week) ($n = 14$)

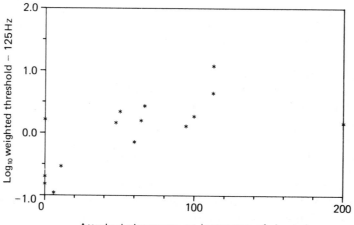

Fig. 5.10 125 Hz baseline thresholds and effect of treatment (attacks during treatment as a percentage of attacks during placebo) ($n = 14$)

THERMAL SENSITIVITY IN RAYNAUD'S PHENOMENON

It was mentioned previously that thermoreceptors sensitive to 'warm' and 'cold' stimuli are present in glabrous skin. The temperatures at which a person will say objects are 'warm' and 'cool' depend on their finger temperature at the time of test. However, the differences between the temperatures for feeling 'warm' and feeling 'cool' remain the same across a wide range of initial skin temperatures (Kenshalo, 1970). Various methods for determining temperature perception thresholds have been used, such as temperature gradients across metal rods or circulated water. One way of generating changing temperature is to use a Peltier heat pump.

The Peltier heat pump is a double-faced semi-conductor device, the surface temperature of which can be rapidly changed by the passing of an electrical current. During the investigation carried out with vibration-exposed workers, and with primary Raynaud's patients, a simple Peltier heat pump device was employed to measure thermal perception thresholds. The Peltier device was mounted on a large heat-sink and its surface temperature was increased and decreased under microcomputer control. The tip of the subject's finger was placed on the head pump and the temperature was decreased at a constant rate. When the plate was felt to be getting 'cooler' the subject responded by pressing a hand-held switch. The temperature was then increased until the subject felt the plate getting 'warmer' at which point the hand-held switch was released. This process was repeated four times and the difference between 'warm' and 'cool' thresholds was recorded.

For vibration-exposed workers, significant differences in temperature difference thresholds were found between persons with VWF, without VWF and non-exposed controls. However, the differences between the three groups were less marked than the differences in vibrotactile thresholds. For patients with primary Raynaud's disease there was a non-significant tendency for thresholds to be elevated above those of the control population (Table 5.2). Thresholds above the 90% point of the control population were found for 5 out of 36 patients (cf. 12 and 7 out of 36 for 125 Hz and 31.5 Hz vibrotactile thresholds, respectively).

The results suggest that sensory loss in Raynaud's phenomenon affects thermal sensitivity as well as vibrotactile sensitivity.

Table 5.2 Temperature difference thresholds (median and inter quartile ranges) for patients with primary Raynaud's disease compared with controls

	Temperature difference thresholds (°C)
Control (*n* = 37)	9.3 (7.3–14.6)
Primary Raynaud's (*n* = 32)	11.2 (8.5–15.6)

They also suggest that this effect is less than that for vibrotactile sensitivity. However, the variation within groups is large. It is likely that measures of thermal sensitivity are confounded by 'noise' from two sources. First, the apparatus used in this study did not closely control the rate of change of temperature; this was particularly the case when low temperatures were required. In the apparatus used by Kenshalo (1970) a complex water-cooling system was employed to alleviate this problem. The second source of variability is less easy to control. Unlike the vibrotactile test which involves a simple detection task (is the stimulus present or absent?), the thermal detection task requires a subjective, semantic judgement as to what may constitute 'getting warmer' and 'getting cooler'. Although such judgements may be consistent on repeated measure from a single person, they will vary from person to person. This inherent variability needs to be taken in to account in the use of any measures of thermal sensitivity.

CONCLUSIONS

The measurement of vibrotactile thresholds provides a clear and simple measure of peripheral sensory function. This function is impaired in some patients with primary Raynaud's disease, particularly where vasospastic attacks are frequent. That vasospasm does not cause elevated thresholds is suggested by the presence of abnormal thresholds on digits other than those liable to vasospastic attacks. It is possible that there is a common underlying mechanism for both sensory and circulatory impairment.

The lack of a clear relationship between elevated thresholds and blanching in persons with vibration-induced white finger may indicate that the underlying mechanisms of these two disorders are different. Alternatively, any relationship between thresholds and VWF may be obscured by the large direct affect of vibration exposure on vibrotactile thresholds.

The authors' studies have indicated that the measurement of vibrotactile thresholds may have a useful role to play in the diagnosis and treatment of primary Raynaud's disease. Its potential use as a predictor of response to drug treatment is of particular interest. As research tools, measures of sensory function, such as vibrotactile thresholds, may be used alongside measures of circulatory function to elucidate the mechanism underlying Raynaud's phenomenon.

REFERENCES

Aatola, S., Starck, J., Pyykko, I., Farkkila, M. and Korhonen, O. (1982) Vibration detection thresholds of lumberjacks. NAS-82 Foredraft, Stockholm, 237–239.

Challoner, V, *et al.* (in preparation).

Geldard, F.A. (1940) The perception of mechanical vibration: 1 History of a controversy. *J. Gen. Psychol.*, **22**, 243–69.

Goldberg, J.M. and Lindblom, U. (1979) Standardised method of determining vibratory perception thresholds for diagnosis and screening in neurological investigations. *J. Neurol. Neurosurg. Psychiatr.*, **42**, 795–803.

Gordon, G. (ed.) (1978) *Active Touch. The Mechanism of Recognition of Objects by Manipulation: a Multidisciplinary Approach.* Pergamon Press, Oxford.

Green, B.G. (1977) The effect of skin temperature on vibrotactile sensitivity. *Perception Psychophysics*, **21**, 243–8.

Griffin, M.J. (1982) The effects of vibration on health. *ISVR Memorandum 632*, University of Southampton, England.

Harada, N. and Matsumoto, T. (1984) Validity of various function tests performed in Japan as a screening test for vibration syndrome. *Int. Arch. Occup. Health*, *SG*, 283–293.

Hayward, R.A. (1986) Vibrotactile thresholds: Reproducibility and frequency function. United Kingdom Informal Group Meeting on Human Response to Vibration. University of Technology, Loughborough, UK.

Hayward, R.A. and Griffin, M.J. (1986) Measures of vibrotactile sensitivity in persons exposed to hand–arm vibration. *Scand. J. Work. Environ. Health*, **12**, 423–7.

Hayward, R.A. and Griffin, M.J. (in preparation).

Iggo, A. (1982) Cutaneous sensory mechanisms, in *The Senses* (eds H.B. Barlow and J.D. Mollon), Cambridge University Press, Cambridge.

Katz, D. (1925) Der Aufbau der Tastwelt. *Z. Psychol.*, Ergänzungsband 11.

Kenshalo, D.R. (1970) Psychophysical studies of temperature sensitivity, *Contributions to Sensory Physiology* (ed. W. Neff), Academic Press, New York.

Knudsen, V.O. (1928) 'Hearing' with the sense of touch. *J. Gen. Psychol.*, **1**, 320–52.

Olsen, N. and Neilsen, S.L. (1979) Diagnosis of Raynaud's phenomenon in quarrymans' traumatic vasospastic disease. *Scand. J. Work Environ. Health.*, **5**, 249–56.

Pelmear, P.L., Taylor, W. and Pearson, J.C.G. (1975) Clinical objectives tests of vibration white finger, in *Vibration White Finger in Industry* (eds W. Taylor and P.W. Pelmear), Academic Press, New York.

Quilliam, T.A. (1978) The structure of finger print skin, in *Active Touch. The Mechanism of Recognition of Objects by Manipulation: a Multidisciplinary Approach* (ed. G. Gordon), Pergamon Press, Oxford.

Rumpf, H.T.M. (1889) Uber einen Fall von Syringomyelie rebst Beiträgen zur Untersuchung der Sensibilität. *Neurol. Zentral.*, **8**, 222–30.

Salle, H.J.A. and Verbank, M.M. (1984) Comparison of five methods for measurement of vibratory perception. *Int. Arch. Occup. Environ. Health*, **53**, 303–9.

Taylor, W. and Pelmear, P.L. (eds) (1975) *Vibration White Finger in Industry*. Academic Press, New York.

Verrillo, R.T. (1966) A duplex mechanism of mechanoreception, in *The Skin Sense* (ed. D.R. Kenshalo), C.C. Thomas, Springfield, Illinois.

Weitz, J. (1941) Vibratory sensitivity as a function of skin temperature. *J. Exp. Psychol.*, **28**, 21–36.

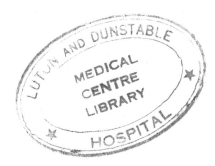

6 Thermographic assessment in Raynaud's phenomenon

RAY P. CLARK

INTRODUCTION

There is currently considerable debate as to the characterization and classification of Raynaud's phenomenon. Symptoms have a great variation in severity.

Some ambiguity exists between the terms Raynaud's disease, Raynaud's syndrome and Raynaud's phenomenon, and between primary and secondary Raynaud's. As mentioned in Chapter 1, the symptoms of Raynaud's phenomenon can occur spontaneously or in association with connective tissue disorders such as scleroderma (systemic sclerosis), SLE (systemic lupus erythematosus) and rheumatoid arthritis. Some of the difficulties of classification are in the main due to problems of assessing the condition objectively. To this end a number of tests are currently being evaluated which are aimed at measuring the finger microcirculation, either directly or indirectly.

Important among these techniques is the use of infrared thermography to characterize Raynaud's phenomenon by skin temperature patterns and to quantify the way in which these patterns respond to hot or cold challenge. This chapter outlines the technique of infrared thermography and discusses some of the findings in patients with vasospastic disorders.

INFRARED THERMOGRAPHY

Infrared thermography produces a 'map' of surface temperature distribution from the energy emitted by the skin in the infrared portion of the electromagnetic spectrum. A special scanner picks up the infrared radiation and the signals are electronically processed to produce a thermal image on a TV screen. Shades of grey, from black to white, represent temperatures from cold to warm and coloured presentations enable specific colours to represent particular temperatures.

Two wavelengths are used for medical thermography; short-wave radiation in the 2–6μm range is frequently used but machines are becoming available using longer wavelengths (8–14 μm). In both of these wavebands there is a good relationship between infrared emission and surface temperature.

It is important to be able accurately to measure the temperature at the skin surface and most infrared systems are now coupled to imaging analysis computers which are able to calibrate thermal images to give an exact measure of the temperature on any part of the skin.

TEMPERATURE PATTERNS

Skin surface temperature patterns are the result of complex physiological and environmental interactions (Clark and Edholm, 1985). These include metabolism in structures deep to the skin surface, the transmission or insulation of heat energy through subcutaneous tissues and the effects of superficial blood flow in bringing warmed blood from deep structures to the skin surface. The skin is the interface between the body and the environment and thermoregulatory energy exchanges at the skin will further modify the temperature patterns.

It is, therefore, important to standardize conditions for medical thermography both in terms of the environment and of the activity state of the patient.

Patients generally equilibrate for a minimum of 20 minutes before a thermographic examination is made. The temperature of the examination room is carefully controlled at a level depending on the particular investigations being undertaken. Our experience indicates that a warm environment of around 26°c is appropriate for thermographic examination of Raynaud's patients.

STATIC AND DYNAMIC THERMOGRAPHY

In many patients infrared thermograms taken after equilibration can clearly identify the areas of the hands (and feet) that are affected. In some Raynaud's patients there may be steep temperature gradients along the fingers which are similar for all digits and affect both hands to a similar extent (Plate 1). In other patients there may be great asymmetry of temperature pattern with some digits apparently well perfused whilst others may be cold (Plate 2).

In the majority of cases the temperature patterns over the hands are only poorly related to the colour changes that are observed in the skin and upon which much of the traditional diagnosis and description of Raynaud's phenomenon is based.

In some patients, the steady-state skin temperatures and thermal patterns can sometimes be similar to those found in healthy subjects, particularly where the 'Raynaud's' effects are intermittent. In such cases abnormalities may show up in response to a challenge stimulus. The thermal response of the hands to mild, hot or cold stress is proving a useful indicator in assessing Raynaud's phenomenon and related disorders and is described in the following sections.

Cold stress test

In those Raynaud's patients where skin temperature over the hands and fingers is significantly above ambient it is possible to perform a cold stress test and thermographically to follow the subsequent thermal recovery (Clark and Goff, 1986).

In this procedure a thin plastic surgical glove is placed over the hand to be tested. The gloved hand is then immersed in water at 10°C (taking care not to allow the water to make the skin wet) for a period of 1 minute. At the end of this time the hand is removed from the water, the glove discarded and the hand placed on a stand in front of the thermal scanner. The scanner automatically records infrared images at pre-set intervals (generally 20 s) until the thermal recovery is complete.

The stored thermal images are subsequently recalled to the image analysis computer and mean skin temperatures are plotted with time. The resulting thermal recovery curves have a number of features which can help characterize the degree and type of spasticity in Raynaud's patients.

In order to interpret such curves it is necessary to compare them with the responses of healthy subjects undergoing similar tests. In a healthy hand there is a characteristic sequence to the rewarming that occurs on both the palmar and dorsal surfaces.

On the palmar surface there is at first a general rewarming of palm to the base of the fingers. Digital vessels then open, allowing blood to flow to the finger tips where the arteriovenous anastomosis (or shunts) open. At this stage the rewarming continues from the base of the fingers distally and the finger proximally. This pattern is very repeatable in healthy subjects and takes place, on average, in some 7–8 minutes although there is a variation in time of response from some 4 minutes to 10–12 minutes. This sequence of events is illustrated in Plate 3 which shows a series of thermograms of the palmar surface taken at 20 s intervals after cold stress in a healthy subject.

When the dorsal surface is thermographically viewed after cold stress, the area under the nail beds warms first and the fingers then heat distally from the base of the nails to the knuckles.

A typical thermal recovery curve resulting from analysis of

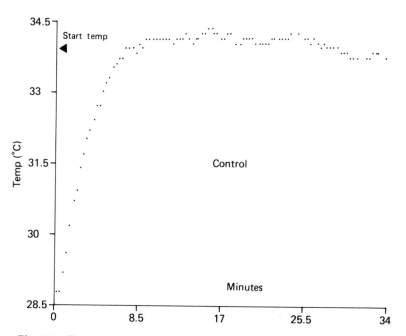

Fig. 6.1 Rewarming curve for the hand (palmar surface) of a healthy subject showing recovery to the start temperature after some 7 minutes, followed by an overshoot due to a degree of reactive hyperaemia

such images is shown for the palmar surface in Fig. 6.1. There is a rapid and progressive rise in skin temperature to the value found before the cold stress; this is followed by an overshoot of temperature due to some reactive hyperaemia. It should be emphasized that the cold stress is relatively mild, unlike those used in some physiological tests where a limb may be immersed in iced water for a considerable time. The mild cold stress of 10°C for one minute has been found to be satisfactorily tolerated by all patients so far tested.

A typical recovery curve associated with Raynaud's phenomenon is seen in Fig. 6.2. There is a very sluggish rewarming which reaches a plateau well before the pre-test temperature is achieved. In many cases the start temperature is not reached even if observation is continued for up to one hour.

In cases where the thermal recovery is asymmetrical and varies in degree and rate for different digits, it is possible to plot the recovery of each digit separately to characterize the rewarm-

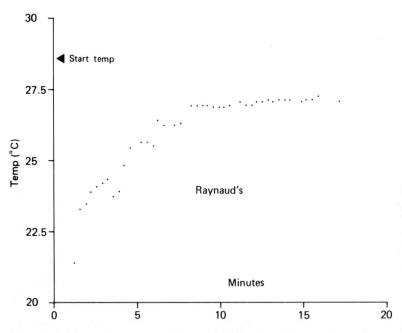

Fig. 6.2 Thermal recovery after cold stress in a Raynaud's patient showing a very sluggish response

ing. This will complement the information that is obtained by simple visual examination of the thermal image sequence.

Hot stress test

In some Raynaud's patients it is not practicable to carry out a cold stress test because the digits are cold with a bland pattern that shows no response to the cold challenge. In such cases a hot stress test often provides much more useful information.

The hot stress is carried out by immersing a gloved hand in water at 45°C for one minute. The glove is then discarded (as in the cold test) and the thermal recovery recorded by the thermographic system.

In some patients the recovery after hot stress is similar to that shown in Fig. 6.3 where the temperature falls steadily to leave the skin at the same temperature as before the stress. In such patients the hot test has clearly done nothing to stimulate

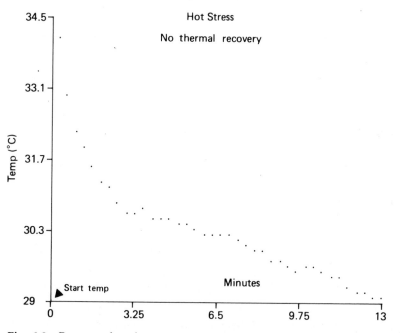

Fig. 6.3 Recovery from hot stress in a patient with Raynaud's phenomenon showing generalized cooling to the start temperature

vascular activity within the digits and there is little potential for the vessels to open and perfuse the tissue.

However, in other patients the response may be similar to that shown in Fig. 6.4. In these cases there is an initial cooling followed by rewarming to a variable degree. The response of such patients is clearly different from those who only undergo progressive cooling. It seems possible to divide Raynaud's patients into two groups, the responders and non-responders in terms of hot challenge.

Those people who respond positively to the hot challenge clearly demonstrate the ability of the digital vessels to perfuse the tissue to some extent. This group is likely to benefit more than the non-responders from vasodilator therapy. Those patients who do not respond positively may be best managed by

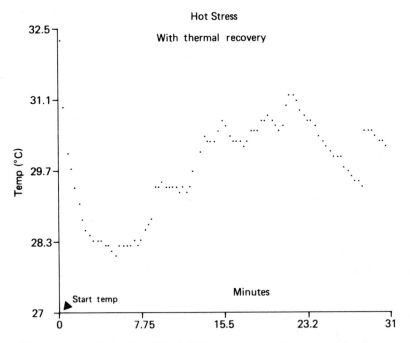

Fig. 6.4 Hot stress in a Raynaud's patient showing rewarming after initial cooling. The thermogram revealed a degree of normal heating after the hot test and demonstrated the ability of certain vessels in the hand to open and conduct blood

advising cold avoidance measures and supplying electrically heated gloves or socks or other heating devices.

SCLERODERMA

The term scleroderma, derived from the Greek, means hard skin. This condition usually affects the hands and feet which become thickened, tough, tight and leathery. When these changes affect internal organs of the body the condition is frequently called systemic sclerosis. Over 90% of patients with scleroderma have Raynaud's phenomenon to some degree and thermography, in association with hot and cold stress tests, is proving useful in assessing these patients.

In scleroderma the thermal recovery curve following cold stress is generally characterized by temperature oscillations superimposed on a general rewarming pattern. Inspection of

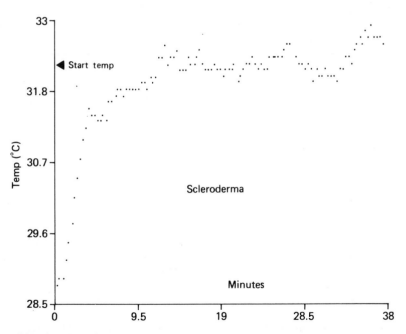

Fig. 6.5 Hand recovery from cold stress in scleroderma showing sluggish recovery to the start temperature followed by thermal oscillations in the hyperaemic phase

the thermographic sequence in such cases shows striated temperature patterns with a patchy and oscillatory nature to the recovery. Figure 6.5 illustrates these oscillations in scleroderma and Fig. 6.6 shows the superimposition of this effect on a sluggish recovery in a patient with both Raynaud's and scleroderma. The presence of such oscillations on a thermal recovery curve in a Raynaud's patient is an indicator to consider the possibility of scleroderma.

The following case illustrates the predictive value of thermographic examination. Plate 4a shows the temperature patterns over the hands of a 14-year-old boy presenting with coldness and stiffness in the left index finger. It was initially thought that some local damage to either the blood vessels or nerves was responsible. Plate 4b shows that the right index finger produced a cooling response when the left hand was cold stressed. Figure

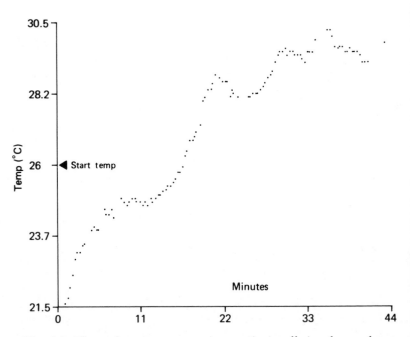

Fig. 6.6 Thermal recovery curve in a patient suffering from scleroderma and Raynaud's phenomenon. The curve exhibits a delayed recovery followed by a substantial overshoot of start temperature, with large temperature oscillations

6.7 shows the thermal recovery curves for the left and right hands and the left index finger. These curves are contrasted with the thermal recovery of the hand of a healthy subject of the same age. From this analysis it is clear that the response of both hands was abnormal with the cold left index finger not adequately characterizing a more generalized condition. In addition, the recovery curves for both hands had a marked oscillatory component.

One year after this thermographic examination this boy was diagnosed as having early scleroderma. The initial thermal findings were clearly indicative of the more generalized nature of the condition than had at first been thought.

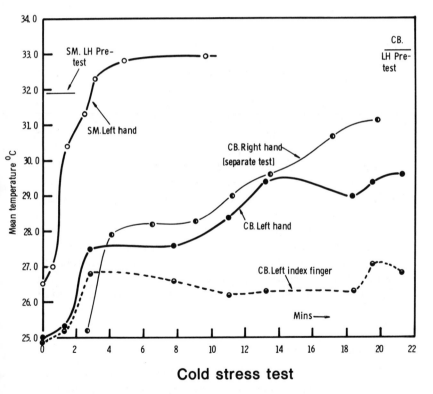

Cold stress test

Fig. 6.7 Thermal recovery of the hands of the 14-year-old boy (C.B.) presenting with a cold left index finger (see text) contrasted with the recovery curve for a healthy child of the same age (S.M.)

ELECTRICALLY HEATED GLOVES

It is often difficult to provide satisfactory treatment for many Raynaud's sufferers and there is now an increasing use of electrically heated gloves to help patients in cold situations. Such gloves have recently also been found to be very useful for the hot stress test described above. Instead of immersing a gloved hand in hot water the patient wears an electrically heated glove for a short period. A particular benefit of this form of the test is that the gloves can be arranged to heat the whole of the palmar surface or simply the fingers. In this way further information as to the responsiveness of the vessels to hot challenge can be determined. Plate 5 shows the temperature pattern over the skin of a Raynaud's patient and the way in which the glove heats the hand.

HIGH RESOLUTION THERMOGRAPHY

Infrared thermography is playing an increasingly important role in the diagnosis and assessment of vasospastic conditions, notably in Raynaud's phenomenon and scleroderma. An exciting new development has been the recent application of very high-resolution thermography to medicine. The Rank Prize Funds have generously supported this development and have produced a comprehensive medical thermographic system equipped with a powerful image analysis computer (Ring and Hughes, 1986). This system produces startlingly detailed thermal patterns as can be seen in Plate 6. Vascular patterns can now be visualized in a detail not possible before to enable more precise differentiation and assessment of areas that may be involved in vasospastic disorders. In addition, this equipment has the ability to visualize individual sweat pores and their secretion activity. This feature will find use in the assessment of sweat function in the skin, particularly in scleroderma.

WIDER USE OF THERMOGRAPHY

One of the difficulties with infrared thermographic techniques over the last few years has been the high cost of the equipment. This has meant that only a few research centres could make full use of the technology. Widespread use by the hospital community generally has been frustrated by both the cost of equip-

ment and scarcity of people experienced in thermographic interpretation.

There have recently been some technological advances in
simpler and cheaper thermographic systems, notably with pyroelectric equipment based on heat-responsive TV tubes. Although
not as sensitive or versatile as the research machines, these
pyroelectric systems, when attached to a microcomputer, can
play a useful role in clinical assessment and diagnosis in the
hospital ward or outpatient department. Recently, some of the
analytical techniques for vasospastic assessment have been
'packaged' in a user-friendly way for use in a pyroelectric
vidicom system (Black *et al.*, 1987). Such equipment, which can
cost about a tenth of that of the research machines can be
expected to find increasing clinical use in the future.

CONCLUSION

Infra-red thermography has an important role to play in the
assessment of vasospastic conditions. The extent and degree of
involvement of various areas can be objectively characterized
and the effect of treatments assessed (Clark, 1987a,b). The
advent of high-resolution thermography and pattern recognition by image-analysis computers is an exciting development
and one that will benefit the understanding of Raynaud's
phenomena and related disorders (Clark, Goff and Jagoe, 1986).

Simpler thermographic systems based on work carried out
with high-resolution machines will make the results of the
research widely available throughout the community.

ACKNOWLEDGEMENTS

Grateful thanks go to M.R. Goff, ABIPP, AMPA, ARPS for
producing the clinical thermograms used to illustrate this chapter.
The author is also indebted to the Rank Prize Funds for making
available the latest high-resolution thermal imaging equipment.

REFERENCES

Black, C.M., Clark, R.P., Darton, K., Goff, M.R., Norman, T.D. and
Spikes, H.A. (1987) A pyroelectric vidicom thermography system
for physiological and clinical use. *J. Physiol.*, **384**, 6P.

Clark, R. (1987a) Thermography: dynamic diagnoses. *General Practitioner*, 20 February, 45–6.

Clark, R. (1987b) Thermography reveals its true colours for diagnosis. *General Practitioner*, 29 May, 57–8.

Clark, R.P. and Edholm, O.G. (1985) *Man and His Thermal Environment.* Edward Arnold, London.

Clark, R.P. and Goff, M.R. (1986) Dynamic thermography in vasospastic diseases, in *Recent Developments in Medical and Physiological Imaging* (eds R.P. Clark and M.R. Goff), Taylor and Francis, London.

Clark, R.P., Goff, M.R. and Jagoe, J.R. (1986) Computer pattern recognition of thermal images, in *Recent Developments in Medical and Physiological Imaging* (eds R.P. Clark and M.R. Goff), Taylor and Francis, London.

Ring, E.F.J. and Hughes, H. (1986) Real-time video thermography, in *Recent Developments in Medical and Physiological Imaging* (eds R.P. Clark and M.R. Goff), Taylor and Francis, London.

7 Drug treatment of Raynaud's phenomenon

DEREK WALLER

It will be clear from the preceding chapters that Raynaud's phenomenon is not a single clearly defined condition. Even the primary form of the disorder may have several underlying contributory causes, while structural changes in the vessels will make a variable contribution to the secondary types. The wide variety of treatments that have been proposed for Raynaud's phenomenon (RP) reflect the uncertainty over pathogenic mechanisms and the unpredictable, often incomplete, response to therapy of individual patients.

GENERAL MEASURES

In secondary RP treatment should be directed, whenever possible, at the underlying cause. Examples are the use of corticosteroids or penicillamine for progressive systemic sclerosis although frequently they give little symptomatic relief for the associated RP. More successfully, correction of hyperviscosity by treating polycythaemia or paraproteinaemia may lead to dramatic responses.

In some situations, precipitating or exacerbating factors can be identified and successfully modified. Occupational vibration-induced white finger is a condition closely related to classical RP which requires a change of job. However, even after removal of the precipitating cause the condition usually persists, although rarely deteriorates further. In other patients, an anatomical constriction may reduce digital blood flow and surgical correction of a cervical rib or carpal tunnel syndrome may be beneficial. Constriction of the subclavian artery by a cervical rib is often associated with a post-stenotic dilatation of the vessel and there is considerable risk of digital emboli from thrombus formed at this site. Surgery should be considered for a cervical rib in the presence of a subclavian bruit even if symptoms in the hands are minimal.

Perhaps the largest group of reversible conditions is that due to drugs. Symptoms may be precipitated by drugs in susceptible patients or symptomatic deterioration of a pre-existing disorder may occur. It is rarely necessary to ask the patient to accept iatrogenic symptoms of RP with the wide variety of effective medicines now available. The beta-adrenoceptor antagonists, such as propranolol, are probably the single most common cause of Raynaud's-like problems. However, in an unselected hypertensive population treated with these drugs, symptoms of RP sufficiently severe to necessitate stopping treatment occur in only about 3–5% of patients. Small scale studies have assessed the effect of giving a beta-adrenoceptor antagonist to normotensive patients with pre-existing RP, and most have failed to demonstrate any deterioration in symptoms or digital blood flow. It may be that normotensive subjects are less susceptible to digital vasospasm with beta-adrenoceptor antagonists than hypertensives. Almost all members of this class of drug block $beta_1$-adrenoceptors, leading to a fall in cardiac output, but with 'non-selective' drugs such as propranolol the loss of $beta_2$-adrenoceptor mediated vasodilatation is probably also important. $Beta_2$-adrenoceptors are mainly responsible for regulation of muscle rather than skin blood flow, but cold peripheries are a common complaint during treatment with non-selective beta-adrenoceptor antagonists. In normal subjects, propranolol has been shown to reduce skin temperature and blood flow in the hands. In contrast, metoprolol which is 'cardioselective' for $beta_1$-adrenoceptors does not alter these measurements and may carry a lesser risk of precipitating RP. Cardioselectivity, however, is a relative property and drugs like metoprolol and atenolol also block $beta_2$-adrenoceptors as the dose is increased. There is rather more convincing evidence that 'intrinsic sympathomimetic activity' (ISA) may reduce the incidence of vasospasm with these drugs. ISA is a property found in highest measure in pindolol, but also in other drugs such as oxprenolol and acebutolol. It results in partial stimulation of beta-adrenoceptors at rest and consequently little change in resting cardiac output or peripheral blood flow. However, the different pharmacological profiles of cardioselective beta-adrenoceptor antagonists or those with ISA do not completely abolish the risk of precipitating RP, and alternative drugs are often required.

Ergotamine preparations, used for the treatment of migraine, are vasoconstrictors which may cause intense digital vasospasm and in overdose this may lead to digital necrosis. They should be avoided in patients known to have RP. Other drugs can also precipitate RP although the mechanisms are often less well understood. These include sulphasalazine (salazopyrine), bromocriptine, methysergide and cyclosporin. There are even anecdotal reports of an association with the vasodilator drug captopril. Clearly the onset or deterioration of RP shortly after the introduction of any new drug should raise the possibility of an idiosyncratic response.

Smoking should be discouraged in patients with RP. Nicotine stimulates autonomic ganglia and the release of catecholamines, promoting vasospasm. This may also reduce the threshold for other provoking factors. Since most smokers regulate their habit subconsciously to maintain their nicotine intake, complete abstinence should be strongly recommended.

NON-PHARMACOLOGICAL APPROACHES TO TREATMENT

Cold is the most common precipitating factor for RP and commonsense measures may be all that are required to reduce the number of attacks.

Simple measures should always be considered before medicines are used. These are considered fully in Chapters 8 and 9.

Active interventions may also be useful. Using a method of 'induced vasodilatation', counterconditioning of digital reactivity may be possible in primary RP. The technique involves immersing the hands in water at 43–45°C while the body is exposed to a cool outdoor temperature, wearing only indoor clothing. This central cooling with peripheral warming is repeated for 8–10 minutes three times daily on alternate days for up to six weeks. Improvement in digital temperature averaging 3.9°C was demonstrated in uncontrolled studies, with benefit lasting up to a year. The repeated hand immersion in water and environmental temperature changes make this a less suitable approach for secondary RP. Biofeedback techniques have also been advocated and are discussed in Chapter 8. A further simple, but effective, manoeuvre was advocated by the American physician, Donald McIntyre. He noticed that skiers warmed their hands by rapid arm rotation down behind the body and up in front of it. The centrifugal force that this generates improves digital perfusion and may abort attacks of vasospasm.

There is some evidence to support the use of transcutaneous

nerve stimulation for treating RP (Kaada, 1982, 1985). A low frequency 2 Hz stimulus is applied to the ulnar edge of the hand and the web between the first and second metatarsal. After an induction period of 15–20 minutes, a stimulus applied for a further 30–45 minutes can raise skin temperature by up to 2°C with a persistent effect for several hours. There is an analgesic effect in addition to cutaneous vasodilatation and preliminary evidence suggests that ischaemic ulcers may heal during treatment. The mechanism is unknown but may involve activation of an axon reflex and withdrawal of local sympathetic tone or possibly local release of vasodilator substances. Unwanted effects of treatment appear to be confined to occipital migraine-like headaches.

SURGICAL MANAGEMENT

Some lines of evidence have suggested that increased sympathetic tone may contribute to the pathogenesis of vasospasm in RP. It is not surprising, therefore, that treatment by sympathectomy was advocated and first reported more than 50 years ago. Very few reported studies have been controlled and it is difficult to evaluate the results. Surgical division of the cervical sympathetic chain is accompanied by a complication rate of about 15%, the most common problem being a partial Horner's syndrome with ipsilateral ptosis or miosis. Neurolytic block by injection of phenol is also used and probably causes few residual complications. The initial symptomatic response is encouraging in up to two-thirds of patients without underlying disorders but even the initial response is poor in those with an underlying vasculitis or obstructive arteriopathy. Longer-term follow up has been disappointing in all groups with a gradual loss of efficacy with time. Thus, there is probably no place for cervical sympathectomy even in patients with resistant RP. Although again there is little controlled evidence, lumbar sympathectomy for RP in the feet may give a more favourable and prolonged response.

PHARMACOLOGICAL TREATMENT OF RP

For many patients, the severity or inconvenience of symptoms may necessitate drug treatment. Alcohol has a vasodilator action on cutaneous blood vessels and may be useful in mildly affected patients, but has obvious limitations. A number of medicines have received a product licence for use in RP but, unfortunately, the evidence for efficacy of several of the older compounds is inadequate and often anecdotal. Nevertheless, for a number of treatments beneficial responses have been demonstrated in well-designed controlled clinical trials. Such trials are particularly important in a condition such as RP. Subjective response to placebo is common and the introduction of bias on the part of the observer or the patient in assessing benefit may give misleading results in open studies. The evidence supporting the use of various drugs is considered below.

Orally active vasodilator drugs

Vasodilator drugs have often received a 'bad press', perhaps largely due to prescribing for inappropriate conditions. Responses will obviously be poor in the presence of obstructive arterial disease as occurs in some forms of secondary RP. In these patients dilatation of healthy vascular beds may shunt or 'steal' blood from the ischaemic tissues. Primary RP is predominantly a vasospastic disorder, and more favourable responses are to be expected. Several drugs with a primary vasodilator action have received attention for treating RP.

Naftidrofuryl (Praxilene)

Both antisympathetic and direct vasodilator actions appear to contribute to the effects of naftidrofuryl on blood vessels. The improvement of oxidative metabolism in ischaemic tissue produced by the drug is unlikely to be relevant to RP. Although several studies have been carried out in RP, the majority have only examined objective responses to a single intravenous dose. Improvement in skin oxygen tension and heat output both indirectly indicated effective vasodilatation with response in about 70% of patients with primary RP. Some patients with secondary RP showed a reduced digital heat output after treatment, suggesting a vasoconstrictor response. Digital vasoconstriction in the hands may occur in healthy volunteers in response to vasodilators, and this finding after naftidrofuryl may indicate the need for caution particularly in the presence of structural change in the digital arterioles. Nevertheless, the limited clinical observations during oral administration have been encouraging, with about a 25% reduction in frequency and severity of attacks and no clear difference in response between primary and secondary RP (Vinckier *et al.*, 1985). Improved finger blood flow has been shown at rest and also following various cold challenges. Unwanted effects do not seem to be a major problem and are usually confined to gastrointestinal disturbance.

Nicotinic acid (Pernivit) and tetranicotinoyl fructose (Bradilan)

Nicotinic acid is a potent direct-acting vasodilator but tends to act preferentially on vessels in the blush area. In therapeutic doses it also causes gastrointestinal irritation and postural hypotension, while tolerance to its beneficial vasodilator action reduces its value further. Tetranicotinoyl fructose (TNF) is a fructose ester of nicotinic acid which is hydrolysed in the alkaline environment of the small intestine, releasing nicotinic acid at a more gradual rate. Tolerance does not seem to be a problem with this formulation, gastrointestinal effects and postural hypotension are unusual, but flushing may still occur. A controlled study in small numbers of patients with RP found no change in the frequency of attacks, but a reduction in their duration and intensity in both primary and secondary RP (Holti, Newell and Poole, 1971). In this and a second single-dose study, the mean skin temperature after cooling the hand and digital blood flow after both local cooling and ischaemia provoked by a sphygmomanometer cuff were improved following the drug. These objective responses were most marked in the primary form of the disorder.

Cyclandelate (Cyclobral, Cyclospasmol)

Cyclandelate acts as a direct vasodilator relaxing vascular smooth muscle and has a product licence in the UK to treat RP. Even in high doses the responses of patients with RP are not dramatic and no controlled evidence has been produced to support its use in this condition. Unwanted vasodilator effects may be troublesome, including headache, flushing and dizziness.

Beta-adrenergic agonists

Isoxsuprine (Defencin, Duvadilan) acts primarily as an agonist at beta-adrenoceptors and increases muscle blood flow in volunteers. The oral formulation is no longer available, and its inability to dilate skin blood vessels suggests that the intravenous formulation should be avoided.

Bamethan (Vasculit), a compound with a similar site of action to isoxsuprine. Again there is only anecdotal evidence to recommend it for RP and similar theoretical reasons why it should be avoided.

Adrenergic blocking agents and related drugs

Many older antihypertensive agents have been tried for RP on the basis of their ability to reduce sympathetic nervous system activity and consequent vasoconstriction. Guanethidine (Ismelin), an adrenergic neurone blocker, is taken up into adrenergic nerve terminals and reduces noradrenaline release. At doses of 30–50 mg daily in patients with RP, finger blood flow in response to cooling has been shown to be less impaired. Unwanted effects, which include postural and exertional hypotension, diarrhoea and failure of ejaculation have made this drug less popular than more modern agents.

Reserpine (Serpasil) blocks adrenergic neurones by depleting their noradrenaline content, and is effective in about 50% of patients with RP, reducing digital vasoconstriction in response to cold. Doses of 0.25–1 mg daily are effective, but in addition to postural hypotension, depression is often reported. Intra-arterial use has been helpful in severe RP and will be discussed separately.

Methyldopa (Aldomet, Dopamet, Medomet) acts in the central nervous system by substituting for the precursors of noradrenaline in the amine synthetic pathway. The weak transmitter produced, alpha-methylnoradrenaline, acts effectively to reduce sympathetic nervous system transmission mainly by an effect on presynaptic alpha$_2$ receptors to reduce release of further monoamines from the nerve terminal. No controlled studies in RP are available, but by using doses of 1–2 g daily, vasospasm was helped in some patients. Hypotension and sedation restrict the use of methyldopa.

Dazoxiben

Thromboxane A_2 is a prostanoid which is produced by platelets and promotes intense vasoconstriction as well as being a mediator of platelet aggregation. Dazoxiben lowers plasma thromboxane A_2 and given orally in pilot studies it alleviated the symptoms of RP. Subsequently, however, two larger trials could not confirm these findings. A further study with a dazoxiben derivative has also provided little evidence of improvement. Dazoxiben cannot at present be considered an option for the treatment of RP.

Ketanserin

Ketanserin is an antagonist at the $5HT_2$ serotonin receptor subtype. Acting via this receptor serotonin is a potent vasoconstrictor and also increases platelet aggregability. Both these actions are antagonized by ketanserin which, when given intravenously, increases skin blood flow and skin temperature in patients with RP. Clinical trials with oral ketanserin have been less promising. A small controlled study using 40 mg twice daily in severe RP associated with connective tissue diseases revealed a response in eight out of ten patients, whereas placebo was ineffective (Roald and Seem, 1984). Recovery time after cold provocation was reduced. Larger studies have been conflicting, some showing convincing benefit (Meloni *et al.*, 1987) whereas others did not demonstrate any advantage over placebo and the place of ketanserin in management of RP awaits clarification.

Nifedipine (Adalat) and related compounds

The dihydropyridine calcium antagonist nifedipine is probably the most widely studied vasodilator in RP. It is an established therapy for the management of angina and hypertension by virtue of its potent vasodilator effects on peripheral resistance vessels and ability to abolish coronary artery spasm. These effects are achieved by limiting the availability of calcium to the intracellular contractile mechanism of vascular smooth muscle. The drug blocks channels responsible for the slow transmembrane calcium flux in response to voltage stimulation. Nifedipine has several other reported actions *in vitro* such as inhibition of platelet aggregation and neutrophil activation, although their relevance to the clinical response in RP is not known. Since the first uncontrolled reports in 1983 of an effect in RP, around 20 large controlled studies in over 350 patients have established its value (Sauza *et al.*, 1984; Corbin *et al.*, 1986; Sarkozi *et al.*, 1986; Waller *et al.*, 1986; Nilsson *et al.*, 1987). As with many other vasodilator drugs, the most impressive results have been obtained in primary RP with at least two-thirds of patients responding, while less than half with secondary RP may receive benefit. Doses ranging from 20 mg to 80 mg daily have been used which probably contribute to the considerable variability in trial results. Nifedipine has a low systemic bioavailability, in other words only an average of about 40% of an oral dose reaches the circulation due to metabolism by the liver as the drug passes through the hepatic portal circulation. This metabolism varies widely between individuals and dose-titration is necessary to achieve an optimal plasma concentration of nifedipine. Most studies in RP report a reduction in the frequency of attacks and in the severity of persisting episodes. In some, but not all, the beneficial clinical effects were accompanied by objective evidence of improved finger blood flow or digital skin temperature recovery time after cold challenge. Healing of digital ulcers in the more severely affected patients has been reported with long-term use, but one study suggested that clinical effectiveness had diminished after 10 weeks of continuous use. Nifedipine increases finger blood flow acutely when given sublingually by biting open a capsule. The onset of digital vasodilatation may be more rapid by this route, which also avoids the initial metabolism of drug in the liver. The potential for on-demand use of this formulation to treat occasional episodes has not been exploited in published reports.

In early studies with nifedipine, the drug was apparently well tolerated but more recent reports have found a high incidence of unwanted effects. These appear to be related to the plasma concentration of the drug and may, therefore, be more frequent with higher doses and rapid release formulations. Although the sustained-release formulations are probably less troublesome, the facial and leg flushing, ankle oedema, palpitations and headaches may still prove unacceptable. Fortunately, many of these do not persist if treatment is continued beyond the first two or three weeks.

Several dihydropyridine derivatives related to nifedipine have been synthesized. All share a powerful vasodilator action, but differ in tissue specificity. Two of these have been the subject of controlled studies in primary RP. Nisoldipine differs from nifedipine in having a longer duration of action and greater vasodilator potency on large arteries. Results so far have been conflicting with one successful study and another failing to demonstrate any benefit, despite a fairly high incidence of unwanted vasodilator effects, similar to those found with nifedipine. Nicardipine (Cardene) has also been studied. In a group of patients mainly with secondary RP, a modest reduction in the number of attacks was produced, while the treatment was apparently well tolerated. A second study in a mixed group of primary and secondary RP, however, did not demonstrate any benefit. There is clearly a need for more extensive evaluations of the many dihydropyridine derivatives now becoming available to determine their relative value and patient acceptability.

Other calcium antagonists

Other calcium antagonists, chemically unrelated to the dihydropyridines (e.g. nifedipine), have been tried in RP. Verapamil was ineffective in a group of 16 patients with both primary and secondary RP but the use of diltiazem appears more encouraging. Using a dose of 60 mg three times daily improvement was first shown in patients with primary RP. The reduction in the number and intensity of attacks was associated with few unwanted effects. Recently this has been confirmed in further studies, with a little over half the patients gaining relief (Vayssairat *et al.*, 1981; Rhedda *et al.*, 1985). In the later studies, diltiazem appeared to reduce the duration of attacks more than their frequency. Unwanted effects with diltiazem are similar in nature to those produced by nifedipine but are less common.

Cinnarizine (Stugeron) and the related compound flunarazine have been less satisfactorily assessed in RP than the other calcium antagonists. Small controlled studies have nevertheless indicated subjective improvement in symptoms with these compounds, maintained over a period of several months. The most common unwanted effects are drowsiness and fatigue.

Alpha-adrenoceptor antagonists

The older alpha-adrenoceptor blocking drugs phenoxybenzamine (Dibenyline) (dose 10–80 mg daily) and tolazoline (25–50 mg daily) were given to small numbers of patients, either as sole treatment or in addition to other vasodilators, and modest benefit was demonstrated. These drugs block both postsynaptic alpha$_1$-adrenoceptors and the presynaptic alpha$_2$-adrenoceptors. The latter regulate noradrenaline release from the neurone by negative feedback and, if blocked, increased noradrenaline release produces a tachycardia. This makes the use of these compounds unacceptable to many and potentially harmful if there is co-existent heart disease. Aggravation of peptic ulcer by these drugs may also limit their tolerability.

The newer alpha blockers such as thymoxamine, prazosin and indoramin are selective for the postsynaptic alpha$_1$-adreno-ceptors and are usually better tolerated. A number of studies with prazosin (Hypovase) using divided doses of 2–6 mg daily indicate an overall response rate of about 60% with little differ-ence between primary and secondary RP patients (Karlberg, Lassvick and Lindstrom, 1981; Nielsen, Vitting and Rasmusen, 1983; Russell and Walsh, 1985). Although doses up to 20 mg/day have been tried, most evidence suggests that prazosin is effective at lower doses and it has a product licence for doses of 1–2 mg twice daily in RP. In some recent investigations objective measurements have also demonstrated improvement in the recovery of finger blood flow after local cooling. Care should be taken to use a small initial dose (0.5 mg) because of the risk of profound postural hypotension after the first dose. Dizziness is the most common adverse effect reported with the low doses usually required for RP.

Indoramin (Baratol) used in doses of up to 50 mg three times daily has produced improvement in both symptoms of RP and objective measurements of blood flow (Robson *et al.*, 1978; Housley, 1983; Wollersheim *et al.*, 1986). Small reductions in blood pressure may occur but unwanted effects, apart from some sedation and dry mouth, were not a problem in the small numbers of patients studied. Subjective improvement has been best demonstrated in a clinical study of RP secondary to rheuma-toid disease. Observations in primary RP are mainly limited to objective measurements of increased finger blood flow after both oral and intravenous indoramin. Clinical responses of these patients were frequently not reported, but were unimpres-sive when mentioned.

Thymoxamine (Opilon) is another potent antagonist at the alpha$_1$ adrenoceptor. Intravenous administration increases skin blood flow in RP, even if cervical sympathectomy has been previously carried out. Oral treatment for two weeks has demonstrated a reduction in number and severity of attacks in primary RP in about two-thirds of the patients. The effects persist with long-term treatment (Jaffe and Grimshaw, 1980; Aylward *et al.*, 1982). Thymoxamine also improved digital blood flow following cold stress in both open and placebo-controlled studies of patients with primary and secondary RP. Minor complaints on treatment included flushing and gastrointestinal disturbances. The recommended dosage is 40 mg four times daily, the duration of action being only about four hours after a single dose; doubling this dose may improve the response in some patients. Dosage frequency is perhaps the most obvious disadvantage of treatment with the drug. Hypotension is unusual since, unlike prazosin and indoramin, it does not lower blood pressure in hypertensive patients.

Angiotensin converting enzyme (ACE) inhibitors

Two ACE inhibitors, captopril (Acepril, Capoten) and enalapril (Innovace) have been used in placebo-controlled studies in RP. They achieve a powerful vasodilatory action by preventing the generation of the potent vasoconstrictor angiotensin II and probably also by reducing the degradation of the vasodilator peptide bradykinin. Captopril in doses of 37.5 mg daily has been the subject of several anecdotal reports of symptomatic relief in severe RP, associated with objective increases in blood flow. Subsequent placebo-controlled study suggested that the drug may be an important treatment option (Trubestein *et al.*, 1984). Experience with enalapril is very limited but doses up to 20 mg/ day were promising in one small study, in both primary and secondary RP. However, it was not found to be effective in a double-blind evaluation in patients with primary Raynaud's phenomenon. Case reports have also appeared claiming that ACE inhibitors may precipitate Raynaud's phenomenon. It is possible that the selectivity of these drugs may lead to dilatation of inappropriate vascular beds in some patients. Despite initial adverse publicity regarding the use of these agents in hypertension and subsequently in heart failure, the use of currently recommended doses in patients with uncomplicated RP should not cause problems. Both ACE inhibitors are well tolerated, with the most common unwanted effects being cough, headache, skin rashes and taste disturbance. If patients are receiving diuretics, small initial doses of ACE inhibitor should be used, preferably after stopping the diuretic on the day before treatment is begun. Further studies are clearly required to adequately evaluate both these agents.

Hydralazine

Hydralazine is a direct-acting vasodilator used mainly for control of hypertension. Anecdotal reports have suggested it may improve digital blood flow in patients with severe RP. It has been used by both intra-arterial infusion for incipient gangrene and orally, alone or with other vasodilators. Its use merits further investigation, although reflex tachycardia may limit its application for long-term administration.

Evening primrose oil

Prostaglandins have given promising results for treatment of RP, but the need to give them parenterally restricts their application. An approach explored recently to circumvent this problem is the use of evening primrose oil. This compound, which contains the fatty acid dihomogamma linoleic acid, is metabolized to vasodilator prostaglandins after absorption. Studies have not so far provided convincing evidence to support its use, with neither clinical nor objective measures showing clear indications of effectiveness.

Topical vasodilators

Topical therapy is an attractive option for the management of RP. Unfortunately, many therapeutic drugs have a molecular size or configuration that prevents transcutaneous absorption. The concept has, however, been tested recently in a limited number of studies.

Topical nitrates

There are several reports supporting the effectiveness of 1–2% nitroglycerine ointment applied to the skin of the affected digits

(Franks, 1982; Nahir, Schapira and Scharf, 1986). Transdermal absorption is rapid and both resting finger blood flow and digital perfusion pressure after cold challenge have been shown to improve, in association with symptomatic responses. Nitroglycerine is rapidly metabolized after absorption and the effects of a single application are short-lived. Problems with headaches and flushing are common. In some studies it has been used successfully in severe secondary RP as an adjunct to oral vasodilator treatment with sympathetic nervous system blockers. It is interesting that despite systemic vasodilator unwanted effects, local benefit only is obtained if the cream is applied to one hand. Tolerance to nitrates in ischaemic heart disease is well recognized if constant plasma levels are maintained, but this phenomenon has not been adequately investigated in RP. Since intermittent nitrate use is likely, concern has been expressed regarding the reports of ischaemic cardiac injury in industrial workers when chronic exposure to nitrates is followed by sudden withdrawal. Although no such problems are known in patients with RP and nitrate doses are much lower, it seems prudent to restrict their use to those who suffer from severe RP and to advise against abrupt withdrawal.

Topical prostaglandins

Many prostaglandins have vasodilator and antiplatelet activities which may be valuable in the treatment of RP. Transcutaneous analogues of these are under development and application of a prostaglandin E_2 analogue (CL115,347, Cyanamid International) in RP has been encouraging (Belch *et al.*, 1985). In patients with primary and secondary disease hand temperature increased, attacks were fewer and shorter, and digital ulcer healing was better than on placebo. Vasodilator headaches and flushing and diarrhoea were reported during use. An important observation was that efficacy was diminished with chronic use, but that intermittent application lessened the likelihood of tolerance occurring.

Drugs with primary rheological activity

The evidence for abnormal plasma and red cell rheology and abnormal platelet aggregability in RP has resulted in trials of drugs whose primary action is to modify these factors. It should be remembered that some drugs with primary vasodilator activity also influence blood rheology, but the relative contribution of these different properties to the clinical response is not known.

Ancrod

Intravenous infusion of ancrod, a product obtained from snake venom, causes acute defibrination and reduces both plasma and whole blood viscosity. Only one pilot study has reported its use in RP and although results suggested it was worthy of further study, the need for parenteral administration and the development of antibodies limit its potential.

Stanozolol (Stromba)

This drug is an anabolic steroid which is used clinically for its enhancement of blood fibrinolytic activity. Hand blood flow was increased by stanozolol in open studies of patients with severe primary and secondary Raynaud's phenomenon, many of whom had failed to respond to cervical sympathectomy (Jarrett, Morland and Browse, 1978). Subjective assessment was limited to questioning the patients about response and a high proportion stated that the attacks were less frequent, shorter duration and less severe during treatment. Fibrinolysis was impaired before treatment in these groups of patients, but although it was demonstrably enhanced by stanozolol, and the plasma fibrinogen concentration fell, whole blood viscosity was unchanged due to a rise in haematocrit. The role of viscosity changes in the improvement of flow with this drug has, therefore, been questioned. Improvement in blood flow and fibrinolytic enhancement were found up to two months after treatment had been withdrawn and it has been postulated that lysis of small vessel thrombi contributes to the therapeutic effects. The occurrence of hirsutism, menstrual disturbance and acne obviously limits the use of stanozolol since the majority of patients with RP are young females. The risk of liver toxicity makes regular monitoring of liver function advisable, even if administration is intermittent.

Inositol nicotinate (Hexopal)

This compound has been shown to have an acute vasodilator action, which reflects its origins as a derivative of nicotinic acid.

Nevertheless, objective studies of the digital circulation have failed to demonstrate any benefit after a two-week treatment period. In contrast, if treatment is continued, progressive improvement in clinical and objective responses have been found after about four weeks, with maximal effect occurring after about two months of treatment (Aylward, 1979; Holti, 1979; Murphy, 1985). After this, increases in resting digital blood flow, and reactive hyperaemia have been clearly demontrated, suggesting that simple vasodilatation is not the major mechanism of action. Various effects have been recorded during long-term administration which may improve blood flow. Fibrinolysis is enhanced, leading to a reduction in plasma fibrinogen concentration and a lowering of plasma viscosity. Serum cholesterol and free fatty acid levels are also reduced and platelet aggregation inhibited. To what extent these longer-term events contribute to the action of the drug is speculative. Using doses ranging from 2 to 4 g/day, up to a 50% mean reduction in attack rate has been reported in several open and one large multicentre placebo-controlled parallel group studies from general practice. All mainly involved patients with primary RP. Responses were not, however, markedly different in the small numbers of patients studied with secondary RP. Unwanted effects during these trials were minor but indigestion was experienced by a few subjects.

Oxpentyfylline (Trental)

This is a xanthine derivative which has little or no vasodilator activity. Its major effects appear to be on blood viscosity and numerous actions have been described. These include improved red cell deformability, possibly by an effect on cell surface calcium, decreased plasma fibrinogen and consequent decreased red cell aggregation and decreased platelet aggregation. The latter effect is through favourable influences on prostaglandin synthesis leading to PGI_2 release from blood vessel endothelium and a decrease in platelet thromboxane synthesis. Despite these potential benefits, there are only uncontrolled reports in small numbers of patients of a beneficial effect in RP and no evidence that the action on blood constituents is relevant to this. The value of oxpentyfylline in RP is consequently not established.

Troxerutin (Paroven)

The therapeutic effects of troxerutin are reported to be mainly due to an increase in red cell deformability. The only pilot study, in seven patients, suggested that it might prove helpful but no larger trials have been published to confirm these preliminary findings. There is, therefore, insufficient evidence to recommend its use.

Ticlopidine

The major action of ticlopidine is on platelet aggregatability, the drug reducing aggregation by an uncertain mechanism. The rationale for use in RP is based on the reporting of abnormal platelet aggregatability in the condition. Despite this, a recent controlled trial failed to find any benefit in patients with primary RP, suggesting that abnormal platelet aggregation is not a major pathogenic mechanism in this disorder.

Parenteral treatment of severe Raynaud's phenomenon

Tissue integrity is only threatened in the most severe forms of primary RP but some patients with a secondary disorder may develop ulceration and infection at the tip of the digit with progression to local gangrene. Severe, intractable RP, particularly if accompanied by digital ulceration may respond best to parenteral treatment. Several approaches have been tried.

Intra-arterial reserpine

Reserpine acts by depleting noradrenergic terminals of their monoamine transmitter. The result is to reduce sympathetic tone and thus vasodilate. Originally introduced for treatment of hypertension, the high incidence of depression and the possible association after long-term use with an increased risk of breast cancer have contributed to a decline in popularity. Following a favourable report in 1967 of intra-arterial infusion in RP, a subsequent study suggested that although the initial response may be favourable with healing of digital ulcers, tolerance rapidly develops. Repeated injections are required, and the major risk is the production of local irritation with permanent arterial damage. This treatment has now been supplanted in many centres by prostaglandin infusions.

Intravenous prostaglandin infusions

Prostaglandins are naturally occurring hormones with a wide variety of actions. Two types, prostaglandin E_1 and I_2 (prostacyclin) are potent vasodilators which also inhibit platelet aggregation. This makes them excellent candidates for treatment of RP, although their use is restricted to parenteral administration. Intravenous infusions of PGE_1, using central venous lines, have been given in controlled single blind and open studies (Clifford *et al.*, 1980; Martin *et al.*, 1981). An increase in pulse volume, improvement in hand temperature and healing of digital ulcers has been recorded after a 72-hour infusion. Symptomatic improvement in these studies was maintained for as long as 6 weeks after the infusion. Other workers have reported improvement in finger systolic pressure after cold challenge. These promising results were followed up in larger studies, one of which gave symptomatic but no objective improvement. The other, a large multicentre study showed no difference between PGE_1 and placebo, both giving similar alleviation of clinical symptoms. Studies such as these emphasize the need for good controlled trials before accepting treatments into established medical practice.

PGI$_2$ has, perhaps, more potential because of its greater potency particularly on platelet aggregation. Once again, infusions of between three and five days duration have produced lasting benefit for up to six weeks (Belch *et al.*, 1981, 1983). Controlled studies with this form of treatment are more encouraging than those with PGE_1 and the advantage of using a peripheral vein make it more attractive. Unwanted vasodilator effects, chiefly hypotension but also headache, flushing and nausea may limit the rate of infusion. Intermittent infusions with slow titration of doses have been used to reduce these problems. A recent open study has also shown that the synthetic prostacyclin analogue iloprost is effective in RP associated with scleroderma. Once again, benefit was observed up to ten weeks after three eight-hour infusions, with healing of almost three quarters of the digital ulcers in the small group of patients studied (Rademaker *et al.*, 1987).

It is not known why prolonged improvement occurs after prostaglandin infusions. Inhibition of platelet aggregation and reduced red cell deformability can be demonstrated for short periods after the infusion, but do not persist as long as the clinical response. An alternative possibility is that white cell function is favourably altered by both PGE_1 and PGI_2, which has well-documented actions on lymphocyte function and neutrophil adhesiveness. At present, however, the role of these actions remains speculative.

Because of the inconvenience of parenteral treatments, it is hoped that oral or transcutaneous analogues of these parenteral agents may in the future provide a more acceptable alternative.

Low-molecular-weight dextran

Dextran must be given by intravenous infusion and primarily acts as a plasma expander. It has also been shown to have several additional actions including enhancement of fibrinolytic activity and reduction of the aggregatability of red cells and platelets. It is claimed to coat vascular endothelium and cellular constituents of blood and thus reduce frictional resistance. These effects will combine to improve blood flow by lowering blood viscosity. Unfortunately, the majority of studies suggesting useful responses are uncontrolled. One controlled study has been reported, which showed clinical improvement and an increase in skin blood flow (Wong *et al.*, 1974).

PLASMA EXCHANGE

Since it requires complex equipment, plasma exchange can only be carried out in hospital-based centres. It is not known how it produces its effect, but many changes occur in the blood during such treatment. The patient's blood is withdrawn and centrifuged to separate the red cells which are then reinfused, suspended in either exhausted plasma from transfusion centres or a combination of fresh frozen plasma, purified protein fraction or crystalloids. Plasma beta thromboglobulin and fibrinogen concentrations are reduced and, as a consequence, plasma and whole blood viscosity also fall. Red cell deformability may be improved and the aggregatability of platelets impaired. Which, if any, of these are responsible for the increased blood flow to the hand that can be demonstrated after treatment remains unknown. Patients treated usually have had either secondary RP or severe primary disease and in some cases the clinical response lasted up to six months after a course of treatment. Healing of digital ulceration has also been noted (O'Reilly *et al.*, 1979; Hamilton, White and Cotton, 1980). Because of the complexity, expense and time required for this type of treatment, trials designed to determine which patients are most likely to respond are required before rational use can be made of plasma exchange.

CONCLUSIONS

The wide variety of treatments proposed for RP is testimony to our incomplete understanding of the nature of the condition. Many patients will respond to commonsense non-pharmacological measures, which should always be tried initially and encouraged even if further treatment becomes necessary. Drug therapy is at present empirical, but oral vasodilators have shown some promise. Up to two-thirds of patients with primary RP and about half those with secondary RP are likely to obtain a response to one or more vasodilators. Comparative studies of vasodilators are almost non-existent but well designed and executed controlled trials have shown reduced frequency and severity of attacks of RP with individual agents. Of these, the calcium antagonist, nifedipine, is the most widely studied although in conventional capsule formulation is often poorly tolerated. Sustained-release formulations of nifedipine are likely to be more acceptable but unwanted effects or failure to respond necessitate alternative treatments in many patients. In this situation, current evidence favours the use of alpha-adrenoceptor antagonists such as prazosin and thymoxamine or the calcium antagonist diltiazem. Less well documented, yet probably worth considering, are the direct-acting vasodilators naftidrofuryl and tetranicotinoyl fructose or the rheologically active drugs inositol nicotinate and oxpentyfylline. The ACE inhibitor captopril looks promising, and has the advantage of being well tolerated, but there is insufficient evidence from controlled studies and it may paradoxically precipitate RP in some individuals. Local transcutaneous treatment is at present restricted to nitrate cream, which should probably be reserved for adjunctive treatment in severely affected patients.

Parenteral treatment is reserved for intractable RP, often secondary to other disorders. It should be considered if symptoms are disabling despite oral vasodilators, if digital ulceration is severe or if there is incipient gangrene.

REFERENCES

Aylward, M. (1979) Hexopal in Raynaud's disease. *J. Int. Med. Res.*, **7**, 484–91.

Aylward, M., Bater, P.A., Davies, D.E., Dewland, P.M., Lewis, P.A. and Maddock, J. (1982) Long-term monitoring of the effects of thymoxamine hydrochloride tablets in the management of patients with Raynaud's disease. *Curr. Med. Res. Opin.*, **8**, 158–70.

Belch, J.J.F., Drury, J.K., Capell, H., Forbes, C.D., Newman, P., McKenzie, F., Lieberman, P. and Prentice, C.R.M. (1983) Intermittent epoprostenol (prostacyclin) infusion in patients with Raynaud's syndrome: a double blind controlled trial. *Lancet*, **i**, 313–15.

Belch, J.J., Madhok, R., Shaw, B., Lieberman, P., Sturrock, R.D. and Forbes, C.D. (1985) Double-blind trial of CL115,347, a transdermally absorbed prostaglandin E_2 analogue, in treatment of Raynaud's phenomenon. *Lancet*, **i**, 1180–3.

Belch, J.J.F., Newman, P., Drury, J.K., Capell, H., Lieberman, P., James, W.B., Forbes, C.D. and Prentice, C.R. (1981) Successful treatment of Raynaud's syndrome with prostacyclin. *Thromb. Haemost.*, **45**, 255–6.

Clifford, P.C., Martin, M.F.R., Sheddon, E.J., Kirby, J.D., Baird, R.N. and Dieppe, P.A. (1980) Treatment of vasospastic disease with prostaglandin E_1. *Br. Med. J.*, **281**, 1031–4.

Corbin, D.O.C., Wood, D.A., Macintyre, C.C.A. and Housley, E. (1986) A randomised double blind cross-over trial of nifedipine in the treatment of primary Raynaud's phenomenon. *Eur. Heart. J.*, **7**, 165–70.

Franks, A.G. (1982) Topical glyceryl trinitrate as adjunctive treatment in Raynaud's disease. *Lancet*, **i**, 76–7.

Hamilton, W.A.F., White, J.M. and Cotton, L.T. (1980) Plasma exchange in Raynaud's phenomenon. *Lancet*, **ii**, 475.

Holti, G. (1979) An experimentally controlled evaluation of the effect of inositol nicotinate upon the digital blood flow in patients with Raynaud's phenomenon. *J. Int. Med. Res.*, **7**, 473–83.

Holti, G., Newell, D.J. and Poole, H.G. (1971) Tetranicotinoylfructose in disorders of digital blood flow. *Practitioner*, **207**, 654–8.

Housley, E. (1983) Indoramin in Raynaud's phenomenon. *Res. Clin. For.*, **5**, 73–8.

Jaffe, G.V. and Grimshaw, J.J. (1980) Thymoxamine for Raynaud's disease and chilblains. *Br. J. Clin. Pract.*, **34**, 343–6.

Jarrett, P.E.M., Morland, M. and Browse, N.L. (1978) Treatment of Raynaud's phenomenon by fibrinolytic enhancement. *Br. Med. J.*, **2**, 523–5.

Kaada, B. (1982) Vasodilatation induced by transcutaneous nerve stimulation in peripheral ischaemia (Raynaud's phenomenon and diabetic polyneuropathy). *Eur. Heart J.*, **3**, 303–14.

Kaada, B. (1985) Use of transcutaneous nerve stimulation (TNS) in the treatment of chronic ulceration and peripheral vascular disorders. *Acupuncture and Electro-Therap. Res. J.*, **10**, 235–6.

Karlberg, B.E., Lassvick, C. and Lindstrom, F.D. (1981) Prazosin in Raynaud's phenomenon. A pilot study with measurements of vasoactive hormones. *Proc. Roy. Coll. Phys.*, **41**, 79–84.

Martin, M.F.R., Dowd, P.M., Ring, E.F.J., Cooke, E.D., Dieppe, P.A. and Kirby, J.D.T. (1981) Prostaglandin E_1 infusions for vascular insufficiency in progressive systemic sclerosis. *Ann. Rheum. Dis.*, **40**, 350–4.

Meloni, F., Transi, M.G., Sciacca, V., De Felice, C., Bagarone, A. and Sciacca, A. (1987) Therapeutic efficacy of ketanserin, a selective antagonist of serotonin ($5HT_2$) receptors in primary and secondary Raynaud's phenomenon. *Angiology*, **38**, 530–5.

Murphy, R. (1985) The effect of inositol nicotinate (Hexopal) in patients with Raynaud's phenomenon. *Clin. Trials J.*, **6**, 521–9.

Nahir, A.M., Schapira, D. and Scharf, Y. (1986) Double-blind randomised trial of nitroderm TTS in the treatment of Raynaud's phenomenon. *Isr. J. Med. Sci.*, **22**, 139–42.

Nielsen, S.L., Vitting, K. and Rasmusen, K. (1983) Prazosin treatment of primary Raynaud's phenomenon. *Eur. J. Clin. Pharmacol.*, **24**, 421–3.

Nilsson, H., Jonason, T., Leppert, J. and Ringqvist, I. (1987) The effect of the calcium entry blocker nifedipine on cold-induced digital vasospasm. A double-blind cross-over study versus placebo. *Acta Med. Scand.*, **221**, 53–60.

O'Reilly, M.J.G., Talpos, G., Roberts, V.C., White, J.M. and Cotton, L.T. (1979) Controlled trial of plasma exchange in the treatment of Raynaud's phenomenon. *Br. Med. J.*, **1**, 1113–5.

Rademaker, M., Thomas, R.H.M., Provost, G., Beacham, T.A., Cooke, E.D. and Kirby, J.D. (1987) Prolonged increase in digital blood flow following iloprost infusion in patients with systemic sclerosis. *Postgrad. Med. J.*, **63**, 617–20.

Rhedda, A., McCans, J., Willan, A.R. and Ford, P.M. (1985) A double-blind placebo controlled cross-over randomised trial of diltiazem in Raynaud's phenomenon. *J. Rheumatol.*, **12**, 724–7.

Roald, O.K. and Seem, E. (1984) Treatment of Raynaud's phenomenon with ketanserin in patients with connective tissue disorders. *Br. Med. J.*, **289**, 57–9.

Robson, P., Pearce, V., Antcliff, A.C. and Hamilton, M. (1978) Double-blind trial of indoramin in digital artery disease. *Br. J. Clin. Pharmacol.*, **6**, 88–90.

Russell, I.J. and Walsh, R.A. (1985) Prazosin treatment of Raynaud's phenomenon: a double blind single cross-over study. *J. Rheumatol.*, **12**, 94–8.

Sarkozi, J., Bookman, A.A., Mahon, W., Ramsay, C., Detsky, A.S. and Keystone, E.C. (1986) Nifedipine in the treatment of idiopathic Raynaud's syndrome. *J. Rheumatol.*, **13**, 331–6.

Sauza, J., Kraus, A., Gonzalez-Amaro, R., Alarcom-Segovia, D. (1984) Effect of the calcium channel blocker nifedipine on Raynaud's phenomenon. A controlled double blind trial. *J. Rheumatol.*, **11**, 362–4.

Trubestein, G., Wigger, E., Trubestein, R., Ludwig, M., Wilgalis, M. and Stumpe, K.O. (1984) Treatment of Raynaud's phenomenon with captopril. *Deutsch Med. Wochenschr.*, **109**, 857–60.

Vayssairat, M., Capron, L., Fiessenger, J.N., Mathieu, J.F. and Housset, E. (1981) Calcium channel blockers and Raynaud's disease. *Ann. Intern. Med.*, **95**, 243.

Vinckier, L., Hatron, P.Y., Mosnier, M., Coget, J. and Devulder, B. (1985) Naftidrofuryl (Praxilene) in the treatment of Raynaud's syndrome. *NPN Medicine*, **5**, 516–19.

Waller, D.G., Challenor, V.F., Francis, D.A. and Roath, O.S. (1986) Clinical and rheological effects of nifedipine in Raynaud's phenomenon. *Br. J. Clin. Pharmacol.*, **22**, 449–54.

Wollersheim, H., Thien, T., Fennis, J., van Elteren, P. and van't Laar, A. (1986) Double-blind placebo-controlled study of prazosin in Raynaud's phenomenon. *Clin. Pharmacol. Ther.*, **40**, 219–25.

Wong, W.H., Freedman, R.I., Rabens, S.F., Schwartz, S. and Levan, N.E. (1974) Low molecular weight dextran therapy for scleroderma. Effects of dextran 40 on blood flow and capillary filtration coefficient in scleroderma. *Arch. Dermatol.*, **110**, 419–22.

8 *Behavioural treatment for Raynaud's disease and phenomenon*

ROBERT R. FREEDMAN

INTRODUCTION

This chapter describes the use of behavioural treatments for idiopathic Raynaud's disease and for Raynaud's phenomenon secondary to scleroderma. The pathophysiological mechanisms of primary and secondary Raynaud's are not known. While Raynaud (1888) hypothesized an overactivity of the sympathetic nervous system (SNS) leading to an increased vasoconstrictor response to cold, Lewis (1929) felt the attacks to be caused by a 'local fault' in which the digital blood vessels were hypersensitive to local cooling. Recent work in our laboratory (Freedman *et al.*, 1987b) has found increased alpha-adrenergic receptor density and/or sensitivity in digital blood vessels of idiopathic Raynaud's patients compared to age- and sex-matched controls. Ambulatory physiological recordings of patients with idiopathic Raynaud's disease have found about one-third of their vasospastic attacks to be stress-related (Freedman and Ianni, 1983a). In contrast cold ambient temperatures alone were sufficient to provoke most attacks of Raynaud's phenomenon in scleroderma patients in that investigation. Regardless of the aetiology of Raynaud's disease and phenomenon, most studies have shown that these patients have lower levels of finger temperature and finger blood flow than normal persons under most conditions (Coffman and Cohen, 1971; Freedman and Ianni, 1983a). Accordingly, most behavioural procedures have attempted to increase blood flow in these patients, either through temperature biofeedback or relaxation techniques, such as autogenic training.

SELF-CONTROL OF PERIPHERAL BLOOD FLOW

The term biofeedback refers to the use of external monitors to aid one in influencing bodily processes previously unregulated by voluntary acts or physiological responses for which regulation has been disrupted by trauma or disease. In all biofeedback paradigms physiological responses undetectable by an untrained subject are electronically augmented and converted into easily discriminable stimuli. Thus, a person may listen to a tone whose pitch varies precisely with skin temperature or watch a light display which informs him whether his heart rate is above or below a particular level. The subject uses this information presumably through an operant learning process to achieve control of the desired physiological response. Ultimately, the response must be regulated in the natural environment without the use of external feedback.

Three controlled investigations (Keefe, 1975, 1978; Keefe and Gardner, 1979) showed that various combinations of brief temperature feedback training and thermal suggestions produced significant increases in finger temperature ranging from 0.8 to 1.3°C. Subjects generally acquired the response early in training and the magnitude of the response was not increased by additional training sessions. Two controlled studies by Surwit, Shapiro and Feld (1976) showed that, while subjects could be trained to reliably decrease their finger temperature (-2.0°C), they could not produce significant elevations when trained to increase it ($+0.25$°C).

For finger temperature self-control to be of practical value it presumably must be replicable without the use of feedback instrumentation. The first study to examine the ability to increase finger temperature in the absence of feedback was conducted by Stoffer, Jensen and Nesset (1979), although they did not examine the ability to perform this task prior to training. Twenty-four subjects were instructed to increase finger temperature using either contingent feedback, false feedback, or no feedback. During five 13-minute training sessions the contingent and false feedback groups produced significant temperature elevations ($+ 0.5$°C). During the post-training test of voluntary control without feedback, only the contingent feedback group could significantly increase digital temperature ($+0.4$°C).

Two studies (Freedman and Ianni, 1983b) were designed to

assess the ability to increase finger temperature without feed-back as well as outside the laboratory and to determine if physiological relaxation is necessary for feedback-induced vaso-dilation. In the first experiment, 32 subjects were randomly assigned to receive six 56-minute sessions of either finger temperature feedback, frontalis EMG feedback, autogenic training or simple instructions to increase finger temperature. During training, subjects receiving temperature feedback showed significant increases in finger temperature during the first 12 minutes of the first session only, an effect not shown by the other subjects (Fig. 8.1). Subjects as a whole showed within-session declines in heart rate, respiration rate, and frontalis EMG level. During the post-training test of voluntary control in the laboratory, only the temperature feedback group produced a significant elevation in digital temperature. In the final voluntary control test, conducted outside the laboratory, no temperature increases were found. Thus evidence for having shaped the response through biofeedback was found upon removal of the feedback as long as subjects were asked to vasodilate in the same environment in which they were trained. It appears, however, that the response was not robust enough for generalization to occur.

It was hypothesized that finger temperature elevations produced during temperature feedback might be time limited or that excessive session length might impede training. Kluger, Jamner and Tursky (1985) also found that feedback-induced temperature increases peaked early in the session and subsequently declined. A second experiment was, therefore, performed in which the sessions were shortened. Sixteen subjects were randomly assigned to receive either finger temperature feedback or simple instructions to increase finger temperature. During training, temperature feedback subjects consistently increased their finger temperature (+0.42°C, $P < 0.05$) while those receiving instructions only did not. Increasing the number of training sessions from six to ten had no effect. Subjects in the instructions-only group showed significant declines in heart rate and muscle tension during training, while temperature feedback subjects did not. During the first post-training voluntary control test, temperature feedback subjects were the only ones who demonstrated significant increases in digital temperature (+0.56°C). There were no group differences on other physiolog-

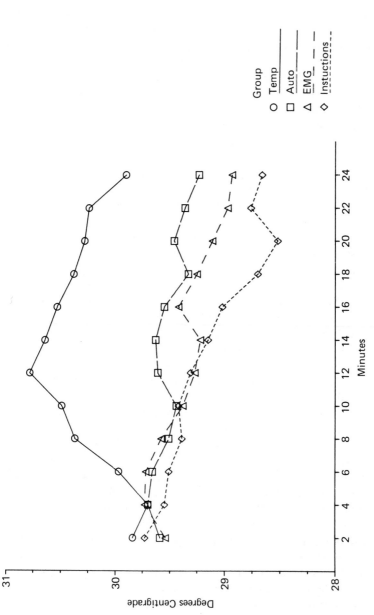

Fig. 8.1 Finger temperatures of temperature feedback, autogenic training, EMG feedback, and instructions only subjects during first training session (From Freedman and Ianni, 1983b)

ical measures. During a similar test performed outside the laboratory with ambulatory monitoring, these subjects were again the only ones to show significant finger temperature elevations. These increases were of substantially larger magnitude (2.41°C) than those produced during prior sessions. Thus, shortening the session length resulted in a robust laboratory training effect and also enhanced generalization of the response to an extra-laboratory setting.

As opposed to biofeedback, considerably less research has been done on the use of relaxation procedures to increase finger temperature in normal subjects. Boudewyns (1976) found significant increases in finger temperature while subjects listened to brief tape-recorded relaxation instructions; these changes were not correlated with measures of skin conductance level or heart rate. Blizard, Cowings and Miller (1975), however, failed to find significant temperature elevations in six sessions of autogenic instructions for hand-warming (tape-recorded phrases such as, 'My hands are warm and heavy').

From the preceding studies it is reasonable to infer that significant elevations in finger temperature can generally be produced by normal subjects using temperature feedback, a conclusion shared by other reviewers (King and Montgomery, 1980). Furthermore, subjects can retain this response over time (Keefe, 1978), and produce it without feedback (Stoffer, Jensen and Nesset, 1979) and outside the laboratory (Freedman and Ianni, 1983b).

Subjects seem to acquire the temperature feedback response within a few training sessions and the magnitude of this response does not increase with additional training (Freedman and Ianni, 1983b; Keefe and Gardner, 1979; Surwit, Shapiro and Feld, 1976). Also, it appears that temperature elevations occur shortly after the activation of feedback and may be time limited (Freedman and Iani, 1983b). Reasons for this temporal limit are not known. It is known, however, that intrinsic myogenic activity exists within blood vessels to maintain constant levels of flow despite varying intravascular pressures (Folkow and Neil, 1971). This autoregulatory phenomenon might act in opposition to vasodilation which is attempted through temperature feedback. The notion of a temporal limit to training is supported by the fact that previous studies reporting significant finger temperature increases during temperature feedback utilized training periods of 15 minutes or less (Keefe, 1978; Keefe and Gardner, 1979; Kluger, Jamner and Tursky, 1985; Stoffer, Jensen and Nesset, 1979; Taub and Emurian, 1976) while studies failing to find this effect used periods of 24 minutes or longer (Surwit, 1977; Surwit, Shapiro and Feld, 1976).

It also appears that relaxation, at least as indicated by decreased heart rate, respiration rate, frontalis EMG, or skin conductance level, is not necessary for the vasodilation shown by temperature feedback subjects. In our first study (Freedman and Ianni, 1983b) there were no group differences in these measures; however, temperature feedback subjects were the only ones who produced significant temperature elevations during any session. In the second experiment, instructions-only subjects showed significant declines in heart rate and frontalis EMG level during training, yet could not raise their finger temperature. In contrast, temperature feedback subjects were able to vasodilate despite small increases in heart rate and EMG. Other studies have not found evidence of physiological relaxation during temperature biofeedback (Stoffer, Jensen and Nesset, 1979; Surwit, Shapiro and Feld, 1976; Taub and Emurian, 1976).

A beta-adrenergic vasodilating mechanism has recently been found in the human finger (Cohen and Coffman, 1981) and shown to underlie some of the physiological effects of temperature biofeedback (Freedman *et al.*, 1984b). This is discussed below in greater detail (see Mechanisms of Behavioural Treatments).

Little evidence exists to suggest that normal subjects can increase finger temperature through autogenic training, although only two controlled studies have examined this issue directly (Blizard, Cowings and Miller, 1975; Freedman and Ianni, 1983b). Vasodilation through other procedures, such as progressive relaxation, warrants investigation.

RELAXATION TREATMENT OF RAYNAUD'S DISEASE

In the first controlled study of behavioural treatments for Raynaud's disease (Surwit, Pilon and Fenton, 1978) 30 patients were randomly assigned to receive either autogenic training alone or in combination with temperature feedback. Half the subjects in each group received twelve 45-minute laboratory training sessions while half received home training and three instructional group meetings. In addition, for a one month period, half the subjects served as a waiting list control group for the other half and then received treatment. All subjects were instructed in a response generalization technique in which they practised hand warming many times each day using visual aids as reminders. Subjects as a whole showed significant improvement in response to a cold stress test and reported fewer attacks after treatment. However, the decline in symptom frequency reported by treated subjects (32%) did not differ significantly from that reported by the waiting list controls (10%). There were no significant differences between subjects who received autogenic training alone and those who also received biofeedback or between subjects trained at home and those trained in the laboratory. Also, subjects' heart rates were significantly higher during the post-treatment cold stress test than during the pre-treatment test. One year later the cold stress responses of 19 follow-up subjects had returned to pre-treatment levels, although reported symptom frequency remained improved (Keefe, Surwit and Pilon, 1979). Questionnaire data showed that subjects did not maintain practice of their behavioural procedures during the follow-up period.

Jacobson, Manschreck and Silverberg (1979) treated 12 Raynaud's disease patients with 12 brief sessions of progressive relaxation alone or in combination with temperature feedback. Patients generally showed temperature elevations during training and rated themselves as improved at a one-month follow-up; however, there were no outcome differences between the two groups. At this point four of the six relaxation patients were given temperature biofeedback. Two years later, 11 of the patients were contacted, seven of whom rated themselves as improved. Six of these seven felt that continued clinical benefit depended on regular practice of relaxation exercises.

TEMPERATURE BIOFEEDBACK

Given the vasoconstrictive nature of the symptoms of Raynaud's disease and the ability of normal subjects to learn to increase peripheral blood flow using temperature feedback, it was logical to employ this procedure in the treatment of this disorder. In one investigation (Freedman *et al.*, 1981) six patients with Raynaud's disease and four with secondary Raynaud's phenomenon received twelve 56-minute training sessions of finger temperature biofeedback. Patients showed significant reductions in reported symptom frequency which were maintained for a one-year follow-up period. Small but significant elevations in finger temperature were found during training and were not accompanied by physiological relaxation.

In a review of the literature on transfer of training in biofeedback, Lynn and Freedman (1979) concluded that 'transfer will tend to be minimal when the training stimulus is non-representative of the population of stimuli to which the response is to be transferred.' Since the Raynaud's disease patient must be able to control finger blood flow in cold conditions as well as in the comfortable laboratory environment, a cold stimulus was constructed and introduced during temperature feedback training (Freedman *et al.*, 1979).

In a subsequent investigation Freedman, Ianni and Wenig (1983) tested the relative efficacy of standard temperature feedback and temperature feedback under cold stress in a controlled manner. A total of 32 Raynaud's disease patients were randomly assigned to receive training in either one of these procedures, autogenic training, or frontalis EMG feedback. Patients were tested for the ability to increase temperature without feedback prior to treatment, after treatment, and one year later.

During training, subjects receiving temperature feedback (TEMP) or temperature feedback under cold stress (TEMPCS) showed significant increases (0.60°C) in finger temperature whereas those receiving EMG feedback or autogenic instructions did not (Fig. 8.2). EMG and autogenic subjects showed significant declines in muscle tension and reported stress, and non-significant declines in heart rate, while the other groups did not. During post-training cold stress and voluntary control tests, the temperature elevations of the TEMP subjects were superior to those of the other three groups. One year later, however, the TEMPCS group showed the best performance (+0.5°C) on the voluntary control test. The change shown by the TEMP group (+0.3°C) was still significant, but smaller than that shown previously. Final temperatures during the follow-up test were significantly related to the number of reported attacks. Decrements in reported symptoms were greatest for the TEMPCS group (92.5%), next greatest for the TEMP group (66.8%), followed by the autogenic group (32.6%) and the EMG group

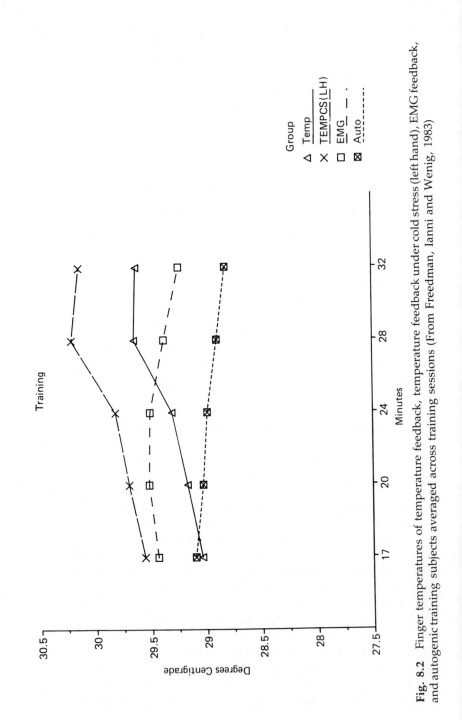

Fig. 8.2 Finger temperatures of temperature feedback, temperature feedback, EMG feedback, and autogenic training subjects averaged across training sessions (From Freedman, Ianni and Wenig, 1983)

(17.0%). During one-year follow-up ambulatory recordings, greater finger-ambient temperature differences were needed to produce attacks in TEMP and TEMPCS subjects compared to EMG and autogenic subjects. Data recently obtained from the TEMP and TEMPCS subjects show that their symptom reductions were retained three years after treatment, although the ability voluntarily to increase finger temperature in the laboratory was lost at the two-year follow-up point (Freedman, Ianni and Wenig, 1985).

Coffman and Cohen (1971) showed that Raynaud's disease patients were most clearly differentiated from normals by low levels of finger capillary blood flow, which might stop completely during vasospastic attacks. Since capillary flow comprises a minority of total finger blood flow and finger temperature is an insensitive measure of blood flow, it seemed possible that subjects might have produced increases in capillary flow that were not detected by finger temperature changes. A subsequent investigation was, therefore, performed in which finger capillary blood flow was measured with an injected radioisotope tracer after the completion of training. Eighteen patients with idiopathic Raynaud's disease were randomly assigned to receive ten sessions of temperature feedback or autogenic training using the procedures of the previous study (Freedman, Ianni and Wenig, 1983). When subjects were tested on their ability to increase blood flow after training, capillary blood flow increased significantly in the temperature feedback group (baseline = 7.8 ± 1.2 ml/100 g/min, feedback = 14.0 ± 2.4, $P < 0.05$) but not in the autogenic group. This effect was retained by the temperature feedback group when they were retested, without feedback, one year later (baseline = 8.9 ± 1.2, voluntary control = 15.8 ± 2.8, $P < 0.05$). These patients are currently being followed for an extended period to determine if capillary blood flow elevations are maintained longer than finger temperature increases.

CONDITIONING PARADIGMS

Peripheral vasodilation can be classically conditioned in normal subjects by pairing external heating of the hands with whole-body cold exposure. Hayduk (1982) first demonstrated this in six normal subjects and found that the vasodilation effect was completely retained when subjects were retested one year later

(Hayduk, 1982). This method has been employed in two studies of the treatment of Raynaud's disease.

In the first (Jobe *et al.*, 1982), eight Raynaud's disease patients and seven normal subjects each received nine training sessions conducted three times per week. Each session consisted of three pairings of peripheral vasodilation (induced by placing the hands in a warm air box) with whole body cold stress at 0°C. Nine patients and seven normal subjects served as no-treatment controls. Treated patients had significantly warmer fingers during the post-treatment 0°C cold stress test than during the pretreatment test. This effect was not shown by the untreated patients or by either group of normals. The untreated patients then received treatment and showed the same vasodilatory effect. Although symptom-report data were not statistically analysed, nine of 16 patients 'reported continued positive effects of the treatment'. A subsequent study compared the effects of this treatment with a combination of frontalis EMG feedback, finger temperature feedback, and relaxation tapes (Jobe *et al.*, 1986). There were no significant differences between the two groups in vasodilation at the end of training or in attack severity or recovery time at one-year follow-up (attack frequency was not reported).

BEHAVIOURAL TREATMENT OF RAYNAUD'S PHENOMENON

The vasospastic attacks of Raynaud's phenomenon are present in a variety of connective tissue disorders such as scleroderma. As in Raynaud's disease, traditional treatments for Raynaud's phenomenon in scleroderma have been unsatisfactory. However, little work has been done on the behavioural treatment of patients having this disorder. Case studies (Freedman *et al.*, 1981; Freedman and Wenig, 1982) showed that scleroderma patients treated with finger temperature biofeedback were able to increase digital temperature and show some symptomatic improvement. This treatment was then tested in a controlled study (Freedman, Ianni and Wenig, 1984a).

Two men and 22 women meeting the American Rheumatism Association classification criteria for progressive systemic sclerosis and having serological tests positive for ANA, negative for RNP, and negative for Sm were used. In addition, all were required to have bilateral Raynaud's phenomenon unrelated to other causes. They were randomly assigned to receive ten sessions of training in either finger temperature feedback, EMG feedback, or autogenic training using procedures identical to those described above (Freedman, Ianno and Wenig, 1983). Subjects receiving finger temperature biofeedback showed significant increases in finger temperature during training and during a post-training test of voluntary control while those receiving EMG feedback or autogenic training did not. These results could not be attributed to group differences in heart rate, respiration rate, frontalis EMG, or skin conductance level. Following treatment, however, no group showed significant decrements in frequency of reported vasospastic attacks. Upon returning to the laboratory one year later, temperature feedback subjects no longer demonstrated significant finger temperature elevations. There were no group differences in data obtained during ambulatory monitoring or laboratory cold stress tests.

These results are in agreement with others which show that general relaxation is not necessary for vasodilation produced during finger temperature feedback. They are at variance, however, with the findings that this vasodilation reduced the frequency of vasospastic attacks in idiopathic Raynaud's disease and suggest that this effect modifies the blood flow abnormality of the primary disorder but not that occurring in scleroderma. An explanation of this discrepancy must await further knowledge of the aetiologies of both disorders. These findings emphasize the importance of differentiating patients with idiopathic Raynaud's disease from those having underlying connective tissue diseases.

MECHANISMS OF BEHAVIOURAL TREATMENTS

It has been shown in normal persons (Freedman and Ianni, 1983b) and in Raynaud's disease patients that the effects of temperature feedback are physiologically different from those of autogenic training, frontalis EMG feedback, or simple instructions to increase finger temperature. Temperature feedback produces digital vasodilation without bradycardia or decreased muscle tension whereas the other techniques do produce bradycardia and lower EMG levels but not increased finger temperature. Recent research has uncovered a physiological mechanism which may explain increased digital blood flow in the absence of decreased generalized physiological arousal. It has generally been thought that vascular control of digital blood flow resulted solely from sympathetically mediated alpha-adrenergic vasoconstriction. However, recently an active beta-adrenergic vasodilating mechanism has been identified in the human finger (Cohen and Coffman, 1981). We have shown that this mechanism is operative during temperature feedback in both normal persons and patients with Raynaud's disease by local beta blockade of the vasodilation with intra-arterial infusions of propranolol (Freedman *et al.*, 1984b). In this study it was also shown that total finger blood flow, measured with venous occlusion plethysmography, increased significantly during temperature feedback in normals as well as patients. Most importantly, capillary blood flow, shown by Coffman and Cohen (1971) to be abnormally low in Raynaud's patients, increased significantly in patients given temperature feedback. Patients and normals given autogenic training showed significant bradycardia but no significant changes in finger total or capillary blood flow.

The only known efferent vasomotor nerves in human fingers are adrenergic; neurogenic vasoconstriction is caused by the interaction of released norepinephrine with post-junctional α-adrenergic receptors. The finding of a β-adrenergic mechanism in temperature biofeedback thus raised the question of whether feedback-induced vasodilation is neurally mediated. We therefore conducted a second investigation (Freedman *et al.*, 1987a) in which the nerves to two fingers were blocked with xylocaine, finger blood flow was reduced with intra-arterial norepinephrine, and the propranolol infusion of the previous study was repeated. In two separate studies of normal subjects ($n = 8$, $n = 9$) and a subsequent study with Raynaud's disease patients ($n = 10$), it was found that the vasodilation produced by temperature feedback was not attenuated by nerve-blockade or norepinephrine, but was reduced by propranolol. Thus, the beta-adrenergic vasodilating mechanism of finger temperature biofeedback does not appear to be mediated through the digital nerves.

COMMENT

Although work on the behavioural treatment of Raynaud's disease began over 10 years ago, relatively few studies have employed follow-up periods of at least one year. This is surprising, since the symptoms are so clearly affected by seasonal variation. The studies focusing on relaxation procedures employed essentially similar methods and achieved similar results. Surwit, Pilon and Fenton (1978) and Jacobson, Manschreck and Silverberg (1979) treated subjects with relaxation procedures alone or in combination with temperature biofeedback and found no group differences in treatment outcome. This is not surprising in light of evidence that temperature biofeedback and autogenic training operate through fundamentally different physiological mechanisms (Freedman *et al.*, 1984b). Thus, the combination of these procedures may impede rather than facilitate self-regulation of physiological functioning. Although the reported improvement in attack frequency in treated subjects in the first study (32%) was significantly different from pretreatment levels, it did not significantly differ from the improvement shown by untreated subjects (10%). These results are not impressive in light of attack-frequency improvements of 25% and 28% in placebo-treated subjects in recent double-blind drug studies (Winston *et al.*, 1983; Wollersheim *et al.*, 1986). The results of the Jacobson, Manschreck and Silverberg (1979) study are more difficult to evaluate since the measure of symptom improvement was undefined and was obtained through a single telephone contact rather than through regular, daily diaries.

Substantially better results were obtained when Raynaud's disease patients were treated with temperature biofeedback procedures in the absence of relaxation (Freedman, Ianni and Wenig, 1983). At one-year follow-up in that investigation, subjects given temperature feedback alone or in combination with local cold stress showed reported attack frequency improvements of 66.8% and 92.5% respectively and could significantly increase finger temperature without feedback. Moreover, they required colder temperatures to produce attacks during 24-hour ambulatory monitoring, compared to subjects given autogenic training or EMG feedback, who had reported symptom improvements of 32% and 17%, respectively. The symptom reductions reported by both temperature feedback groups were retained two and three years later although the ability to increase finger temperature in the laboratory was lost at the two-year follow-up point (Freedman, Ianni and Wenig, 1985). A subsequent study (Freedman *et al.*, 1987a) found that Raynaud's disease patients given temperature feedback could voluntarily increase finger capillary blood flow and retained this effect one year later. This is important because capillary blood flow supplies oxygen to the surrounding tissue and is most abnormally depressed in Raynaud's patients (Coffman and Cohen, 1971). The only controlled study of behavioural treatments for Raynaud's phenomenon in scleroderma (Freedman, Ianni and Wenig, 1984a) found no long-term effects for any group, suggesting that with current methods, behavioural treatments are unable to modify the blood flow abnormalities in that disease.

The use of conditioned vasodilation with Raynaud's disease is intriguing in light of Hayduk's (1982) demonstration that normal subjects retained this effect for one year. The two investigations of this paradigm with Raynaud's patients did not test for retention of this effect at follow-up, did not report attack frequency, and did not assess symptoms with daily diaries (Jobe *et al.*, 1982, 1986).

In conclusion, the strongest evidence for the behavioural treatment of Raynaud's disease comes from studies employing finger temperature biofeedback without relaxation procedures. The results of these studies are consistent, but come from the same laboratory and should be independently replicated. In contrast, there is little evidence at the present time to support the long-term effectiveness of relaxation treatments, alone or in combination with temperature feedback. No study has demonstrated significant physiological effects at one year follow-up and reported attack frequencies do not significantly differ from those of untreated patients. Follow-up data on conditioned vasodilation are insufficient to judge its effectiveness in Raynaud's disease, although Hayduk's (1982) study suggests that further research might be fruitful.

PRACTICAL CONSIDERATIONS

We have identified several procedural variables which are important in the production of voluntary vasodilation with temperature feedback. Since skin temperature is affected by ambient temperature, it is important that the evaluation and training of subjects be conducted in a temperature-controlled room. We have employed an ambient temperature of 23°C in our investigations. Subjects are typically seated in a large armchair with their

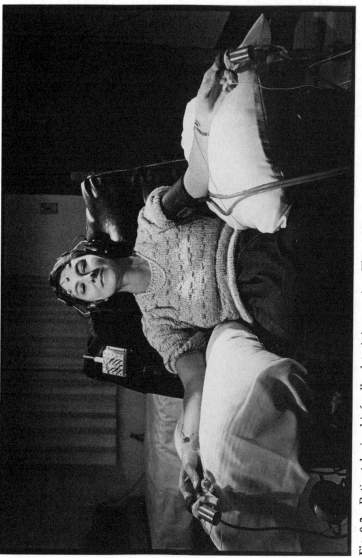

Fig. 8.3 Patient during biofeedback training session. Thermistors are taped to distal end of third fingers; plethysmograph cups and occlusion cuffs are attached to second fingers

hands and arms slightly above heart level (Fig. 8.3). They are instructed to avoid physical manoeuvres such as hand movements and respiratory changes during the recording period. It is important that subjects be physiologically adapted to the laboratory prior to the initiation of training in order to reduce spontaneous fluctuations in skin temperature and blood flow. However, if sessions are made too long, subjects are likely to become bored. We have found that a resting baseline period of 16 minutes followed by a 16-minute training period generally accommodates both factors. Ten sessions are generally administered on a biweekly basis.

Since temperature elevations often occur within a short period of time after the initiation of feedback, it is important that training sessions be brief to reduce subsequent frustration. Many subjects will initially try too hard to perform the temperature feedback task, resulting in vasoconstriction rather than vasodilation. Patients should therefore be dissuaded from focusing excessive attention on the feedback stimulus. Although biofeedback equipment manufacturers have developed elaborate and expensive feedback displays, the specific form of the feedback stimulus is probably not important. However, the stimulus should be neither startling nor intrusive, so that it can be maintained in the periphery of the patient's attention. Coaching the patient to avoid cold-related cognitions may facilitate vasodilation, in addition to reassurance that most patients learn to master the task despite its difficulty. Since finger temperature is affected by ambient temperature, it is important that training be conducted in a room whose temperature is reasonably well-controlled. Spurious fluctuations of room temperature would only increase the difficulty of the temperature feedback task. After the voluntary vasodilation task has been acquired, the gradual introduction of cold stress during training should improve the robustness of the vasodilation response in cold situations outside the laboratory. Patients should be instructed to practise this response when it is opportune to do so. However, we have not found rigid home practice requirements to be beneficial in training.

ACKNOWLEDGEMENT

Research conducted by the author was supported by research grants HL-23828 and HL-30604 from the National Heart, Lung and Blood Institute.

REFERENCES

Blizard, D.A., Cowings, P. and Miller, N.E. (1975) Visceral responses to opposite types of autogenic-training imagery. *Biol. Psychol.*, **3**, 49–55.

Boudewyns, P. (1976) A comparison of the effects of stress: 5. Relaxation instruction on the finger temperature response. *Behav. Ther.*, **7**, 54–67.

Coffman, J. and Cohen, A. (1971) Total and capillary fingertip blood flow in Raynaud's phenomenon. *N. Engl. J. Med.*, **285**, 259–63.

Cohen, R. and Coffman, J. (1981) Beta-Adrenergic vasodilator mechanism in the finger. *Circ. Res.*, **49**, 1196–201.

Folkow, B. and Neil, E. (1971) *Circulation*. Oxford University Press, London.

Freedman, R. and Ianni, P. (1983a) Role of cold and emotional stress in Raynaud's disease and scleroderma. *Br. Med. J.*, **287**, 1499–502.

Freedman, R. and Ianni, P. (1983b) Self-control of digital temperature: physiological factors and transfer effects. *Psychophysiol.*, **20**, 682–8.

Freedman, R., Ianni, P., Hale, P. and Lynn, S. (1979) Treatment of Raynaud's phenomenon with biofeedback and cold desensitization. *Psychophysiol.*, **16**, 182 (Abstract).

Freedman, R., Ianni, P. and Wenig, P. (1983) Behavioural treatment of Raynaud's disease. *J. Cons. Clin. Psychol.*, **51**, 539–49.

Freedman, R., Ianni, P. and Wenig, P. (1984a) Behavioural treatment of Raynaud's phenomenon in scleroderma. *J. Behav. Med.*, **7**, 343–53.

Freedman, R., Ianni, P. and Wenig, P. (1985) Behavioural treatment of Raynaud's disease: long-term followup. *J. Cons. Clin. Psychol.*, **53**, 136.

Freedman, R., Lynn, S., Ianni, P. and Hale, P. (1981) Biofeedback treatment of Raynaud's disease and phenomenon. *Biofeedback Self-Regul.*, **6**, 355–65.

Freedman, R., Sabharwal, S., Ianni, P., Desai, N., Wenig, P. and Mayes, M. (1987a) Non-neural mediation of temperature biofeedback. Paper presented at meeting of the Biofeedback Society of America, Boston, March, 1987.

Freedman, R., Sabharwal, S., Ianni, P. and Wenig, P. (1984b) Beta-Adrenergic vasodilating mechanism in temperature feedback. *Psychophysiol.*, **21**, 577–8.

Freedman, R., Sabharwal, S., Wenig, P. and Mayes, M. (1987b) Increased alpha-adrenergic responsiveness in Raynaud's disease. Paper presented at meeting of the Society for Behavioural Medicine, Washington, DC, March, 1987.

Freedman, R. and Wenig, P. (1982) Pathophysiology and behavioural treatment of scleroderma, in *Behavioral Treatment of Disease* (eds R. Surwit, R. Williams, A. Steptoe and J. Biersner), Plenum, New York, pp. 101–13.

Hayduk, A. (1982) The persistence and transfer of voluntary hand-warming in natural and laboratory settings after one year. *Biofeedback Self-Regul.*, **7**, 49–52.

Jacobson, A., Manschreck, T. and Silverberg, E. (1979) Behavioural treatment for Raynaud's disease: A comparative study with long-term follow-up. *Am. J. Psychiat.*, **136**, 844–6.

Jobe, J., Sampson, J., Roberts, D. and Beetham, W. (1982) Induced vasodilation as treatment for Raynaud's disease. *Ann. Int. Med.*, **97**, 706–9.

Jobe, J., Sampson, J., Roberts, D. and Kelley, J. (1986) Comparison of behavioural treatments for Raynaud's disease. *J. Behav. Med.*, **9**, 89–96.

Keefe, F. (1975) Conditioning changes in differential skin temperature. *Percept. Mot. Skills*, **40**, 283–8.

Keefe, F. (1978) Biofeedback vs. instructional control of skin temperature. *J. Behav. Med.*, **1**, 323–35.

Keefe, F. and Gardner, E. (1979) Learned control of skin temperature: effects of short and long-term biofeedback training. *Behav. Ther.*, **10**, 202–10.

Keefe, F., Surwit, R. and Pilon, R. (1979) A 1-year follow-up of Raynaud's patients treated with behavioural therapy techniques. *J. Behav. Med.*, **2**, 385–91.

King, N.J. and Montgomery, R.B. (1980) Biofeedback induced control of human peripheral temperature: A critical review of the literature. *Psych. Bull.*, **88**, 738–52.

Kluger, M.A., Jamner, L.D. and Tursky, B. (1985) Comparison of the effectiveness of biofeedback and relaxation training on hand warming. *Psychophysiol.*, **22**, 162–6.

Lewis, T. (1929) Experiments relating to the peripheral mechanism involved in spasmodic arrest of circulation in the fingers, a variety of Raynaud's disease. *Heart*, **15**, 7–101.

Lynn, S. and Freedman, R. (1979) Transfer and evaluation of biofeedback treatment, in *Maximizing Treatment Gains – Transfer Enhancement in Psychotherapy* (eds A. Goldstein and F. Kanfer), Academic Press, New York, pp. 445–84.

Raynaud, M. (1888) *New Research on the Nature and Treatment of Local Asphyxia of the Extremities* (Trans. T. Barlow), The New Sydenham Society, London.

Stoffer, G.R., Jensen, J.A.S. and Nesset, B.L. (1979) Effects of contingent versus yoked temperature feedback on voluntary temperature control and cold stress tolerance. *Biofeedback Self-Regul.*, **4**, 51–61.

Surwit, R. (1977) Simple versus complex feedback displays in the training of digital temperature. *J. Cons. Clin. Psychol.*, **45**, 146–7.

Surwit, R., Pilon, R. and Fenton, C. (1978) Behavioral treatment of Raynaud's disease. *J. Behav. Med.*, **1**, 323–35.

Surwit, R.S., Shapiro, D. and Feld, J.L. (1976) Digital temperature autoregulation and associated cardiovascular changes. *Psychophysiol.*, **13**, 242–8.

Taub, E. and Emurian, C.S. (1976) Feedback-aided self-regulation of skin temperature and single feedback locus. *Biofeedback Self-Regul.*, **1**, 147–68.

Winston, E., Pariser, K., Miller, K., Salem, D. and Craeger, M. (1983) Nifedipine as a therapeutic modality for Raynaud's phenomenon. *Arthr. Rheum.*, **26**, 1177–80.

Wollersheim, H., Thien, T., Fennis, J., van Elteren, P. and van't Laar, A. (1986) Double-blind, placebo-controlled study of prazosin in Raynaud's phenomenon. *Clin. Pharmacol. Ther.*, **40**, 219–25.

9 *Keeping warm*

ANNE H. MAWDSLEY

In addition to the treatments mentioned in a previous chapter warm clothing is essential. It is most important to keep the trunk warm to protect the main organs of the body. Several thin layers of clothing should be recommended rather than one thick layer, as the air trapped between the layers will help to insulate the body. A considerable amount of heat is lost from the head area so importance should be given to keeping the head, nose, mouth and face protected from the cold.

Thermal clothing is advisable. Tight clothing should be avoided as this may restrict the blood flow. Hands and feet need adequate covering with the many mittens, gloves and footwear which are available. For those who have problems with their feet, 'comfort' shoes can be prescribed through a hospital.

HEATING AIDS

There are a number of ingenious heating aids which are available.

Thermogel hotmates

These come in different sizes and are small re-usable packs, activated by the press of a button. Once activated the pack becomes very warm as the contents change from being liquid to a solid form. It helps to move the pack around in the hands to make it more supple. The useful heat, according to the type of pack used, can be extended from 45 minutes to 4–5 hours. After use it can be returned to its original state by boiling in a pan of water. Each pack can be used over and over again. This is a very effective way of producing safe heat where and when required. Hotmates are neither toxic nor cause dermatitis.

Charcoal handwarmers

These are easy to use and each stick of charcoal lasts for about 8 hours. A tip for lighting the charcoal is to light a candle first and use the candle to ignite the stick.

Chemical handwarmers

These are small sachets which resemble a tea bag. To operate this portable heat source, simply remove the sachet from the pack, squeeze and expose to the air. They can then be insulated in a pocket or gloves. The small hand and foot warmers last for up to 6 hours and the larger size body warmers for approximately 20 hours. These warm packs are ideal if your heating fails or for taking on either short journeys or a day out.

Body warmers

These are disc-shaped and designed to be worn around the neck or can be put on one's lap when sitting in a chair or wheelchair and remain hot for 3 hours. They can be used instead of a hot water bottle in bed, retaining heat for even longer than the 3 hours stated. To recharge just plug into the mains electricity for 4 minutes with the charger provided. They are very efficient, effective and safe.

Electric footmuffs

These are very economical and give a safe, gentle heat. Available from department stores and catalogues.

Electrically heated gloves and socks

Many patients have found considerable benefit from Medmek Electrically Heated Gloves and Socks. These are available on the NHS if prescribed by a hospital consultant in Britain and ordered as a surgical appliance. The gloves and socks run from a small rechargeable battery worn around the waist. The wires are concealed when worn under a coat or jacket. They can also be purchased directly from Medmek Limited, PO Box 18, Romsey, Hants. SO51 9ZX, UK.

Further information on the items mentioned in this chapter and details of membership are available from The Raynaud's Association, 112 Crewe Road, Alsager, Cheshire ST7 2JA, UK.

Appendix: Raynaud's Association Publications

The following publications are available from The Raynaud's Association. If you wish to order copies please send a cheque made payable to 'THE RAYNAUD'S ASSOCIATION' at 112 Crewe Road, Alsager, Cheshire ST7 2JA, England.

Raynaud's – A Better Understanding
by K. Lafferty, MS, FRCS
This book is intended to give a better understanding of the condition and is a factual account of the history and presently accepted theories with regard to its causes and treatment. Price £4.50

Raynaud's – A Handbook for Patients
by Anne H. Mawdsley
Price 70p

Scleroderma – A Handbook for Patients
by Anne H. Mawdsley
Price £1.00

These are booklets for patients containing advice, tips, questions and answers on how to cope with the condition.

Raynaud's – There Are More Questions Than Answers
by Anne H. Mawdsley
Price £1.75
This booklet contains over 100 questions and answers on Raynaud's, scleroderma and other associated conditions.

Prices include postage in the UK. Overseas mailing – Please note the price of Mr Lafferty's book is £6 (Sterling) and also add 50p for each of the handbooks, due to the high cost of postage overseas.

Index